Self-Assessment

Small Animal Soft Tissue Surgery

Second Edition

Kelley M Thieman Mankin
DVM, MS, Dipl ACVS-SA
Department of Small Animal Clinical Sciences
College of Veterinary Medicine
Texas A&M University
College Station, TX, USA

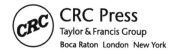

CRC Press
Taylor & Francis Group
Boca Raton London New York

CRC Press is an imprint of the
Taylor & Francis Group, an **informa** business

CRC Press
Taylor & Francis Group
6000 Broken Sound Parkway NW, Suite 300
Boca Raton, FL 33487-2742

Printed on acid-free paper
Version Date: 20140722

International Standard Book Number-13: 978-1-4822-2538-9 (Paperback)

Visit the Taylor & Francis Web site at
http://www.taylorandfrancis.com

and the CRC Press Web site at
http://www.crcpress.com

Preface

This book provides a broad overview of small animal soft tissue surgery. The information is presented in a question and answer format. The answers are of sufficient length to provide detail on the topic at hand. The questions presented in this book should appeal to veterinary students, general practitioners, surgical residents and specialists with an interest in soft tissue surgery. The topics are presented as clinical cases in order for readers to consider the topic and test their knowledge.

The questions in this book were provided by an international group of veterinarians, dedicated to advancing our profession and teaching the art and science of surgery. The contributors have made an effort to make this book thorough and up to date, but the reader should be aware that soft tissue surgery has some controversial topics and alternative answers to some questions do exist.

I enjoyed the writing of this book; my hope is that you enjoy the book and learn from it. This book was written to encourage knowledge. It was written with the hope that readers will strive to understand the act of surgery, but also strive to understand medical and surgical decisions regarding diagnostics and perioperative care of small animals.

Kelley M Thieman Mankin

Contributors

Carobbi Barbara, DVM
Department of Animal Clinical
Medicine, College of Veterinary
Medicine,
Padua University,
Padua, Italy

Alastair Coomer, BVSC, MS, Dipl
ACVS
Veterinary Specialists Group,
Mt Albert, New Zealand

Laura C Cuddy, MVB, MS, Dipl
ACVS-SA
Department of Surgery, Section of
Veterinary Clinical Studies, School
of Agriculture, Food Science and
Veterinary Medicine, University
College Dublin,
Dublin, Ireland

Alison B Diesel, DVM, Dipl ACVD
Department of Small Animal Clinical
Sciences, College of Veterinary
Medicine, Texas A&M University,
College Station, TX, USA

April M Durant, DVM, Dipl ACVS-
SA
Department of Clinical Sciences,
College of Veterinary Medicine,
Kansas State University,
Manhattan, KS, USA

Gary W Ellison, DVM, MS, Dipl
ACVS
Department of Small Animal Clinical
Sciences, College of Veterinary
Medicine, University of Florida,
Gainesville, FL, USA

Katy Fryer, DVM, Dipl ACVS-SA
Sacramento Veterinary Referral
Center,
Sacramento, CA, USA

Ashley E Jones, DVM
Department of Small Animal Clinical
Sciences, College of Veterinary
Medicine, University of Florida,
Gainesville, FL, USA

Kristin Kirkby Shaw, DVM, MS, PhD,
Dipl ACVS, Dipl ACVSMR
Novartis Animal Health US, Inc.,
Greensboro, NC, USA

Elizabeth S Lechner, DVM, Dipl
ACVIM (Internal Medicine)
Palm Beach Veterinary Specialists,
West Palm Beach, FL, USA

Jessica J Leeman, DVM
Seattle Veterinary Specialists,
Kirkland, WA, USA

Gwendolyn J Levine, DVM, Dipl
ACVP (Clinical Pathology)
Department of Veterinary
Pathobiology, College of Veterinary
Medicine & Biomedical Sciences,
Texas A&M University,
College Station, TX, USA

Mauricio Loría Lépiz, DVM, MS, Dipl
ACVA
Department of Small Animal Clinical
Sciences, College of Veterinary
Medicine, Texas A&M University,
College Station, TX, USA

Herbert W Maisenbacher, III, VMD,
Dipl ACVIM (Cardiology)
Veterinary Heart Care,
Virginia Beach, VA, USA

Joseph M Mankin, DVM, Dipl ACVIM (Neurology)
Department of Small Animal Clinical Sciences, College of Veterinary Medicine, Texas A&M University, College Station, TX, USA

Michael B Mison, DVM, Dipl ACVS
Seattle Veterinary Specialists, Kirkland, WA, USA
University of Washington School of Medicine, Department of Comparative Medicine, Seattle, WA, USA

Lysimachos G Papazoglou, DVM, PhD, Member of the Royal College of Veterinary Surgeons
Department of Clinical Sciences, Faculty of Veterinary Medicine, Aristotle University of Thessaloniki, Thessaloniki, Greece

Laura E Peycke, DVM, MS, Dipl ACVS
Department of Small Animal Clinical Sciences, College of Veterinary Medicine, Texas A&M University, College Station, TX, USA

Marije Risselada, DVM, PhD, Dipl ECVS, Dipl ACVS-SA
Department of Clinical Sciences, College of Veterinary Medicine, North Carolina State University, Raleigh, NC, USA

Valery F Scharf, DVM, MS
Department of Small Animal Clinical Sciences, College of Veterinary Medicine, University of Florida, Gainesville, FL, USA

Ameet Singh, BSc, DVM, DVSc, Dipl ACVS
Department of Clinical Studies, Ontario Veterinary College, University of Guelph, Guelph, ON, Canada

Carlos H de M. Souza, Medico Veterinario, MS, Dipl ACVS-SA, Dipl ACVIM (Oncology)
Department of Small Animal Clinical Sciences, College of Veterinary Medicine, University of Florida, Gainesville, FL, USA

Tige H Witsberger, DVM, Dipl ACVS
Mission Veterinary Specialists, San Antonio, TX, USA

Abbreviations

ACDO	Amplatz canine ductal occluder	IFM	immunofluorescent microscopy
ACh	acetylcholine	IV	intravenous
ALP	alkaline phosphatase	LRS	lactated Ringer's solution
ALT	alanine aminotransferase	MG	myasthenia gravis
AST	aspartate aminotransferase	MLO	multilobular osteochondrosarcoma
ATPase	adenosine triphosphatase	MRI	magnetic resonance imaging
AV	atrioventricular	MS	molar substitution
BMBT	buccal mucosal bleeding time	MST	median survival time
BUN	blood urea nitrogen	MW	molecular weight
CBC	complete blood count	OLV	one lung ventilation
CHF	congestive heart failure	PAF	perianal fistula
COP	colloid osmotic pressure	PCV	packed cell volume
CRI	constant rate infusion	PDA	patent ductus arteriosus
CRT	capillary refill time	PFA	platelet function assays
CT	computed tomography	PPDH	peritoneopericardial diaphragmatic hernia
CVD	chronic valvular disease	PPI	proton pump inhibitor
DDAVP	desmopressin acetate	PTFE	polytetrafluoroethylene
DES	diethylstilbestrol	PTH	parathyroid hormone
DNA	deoxyribonucleic acid	RBC	red blood cell
ECG	electrocardiogram	RER	resting energy requirement
ELISA	enzyme-linked immunosorbent assay	RNA	ribonucleic acid
EM	electron microscopy	TCC	transitional cell carcinoma
EMG	electromyography	TECABO	total ear canal ablation with bulla osteotomy
FB	foreign body	TP	total protein
FNA	fine needle aspiration	USMI	urethral sphincter mechanism incompetence
FSI	fronto-sagittal index	VAC	vacuum assisted closure
GDV	gastric dilatation and volvulus	VI	vertebral index
GFR	glomerular filtration rate	VPC	ventricular premature contraction
GIA	gastrointestinal anastomosis	VWD	von Willebrand disease
GMS	Gomori methenamine silver	VWF	von Willebrand factor
GOLPP	geriatric onset laryngeal paralysis polyneuropathy	WBC	white blood cell
HTC	hematocrit		

Classification of cases

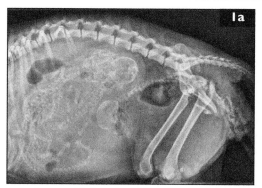

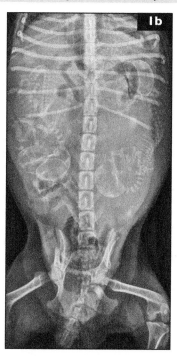

1 A 4-year-old female Chihuahua presents for suspected dystocia. The dog was mated twice; 67 days ago and 65 days ago. The dog has been experiencing strong contractions for the last 45 minutes. Based on ultrasonographic examination, one fetus is dead and the second has a slow heart rate.
i. What is the reason for the inability to whelp (1a, b)?
ii. What surgery do you recommend?
iii. What anesthetic protocol will you use?

2 A 1.5-year-old spayed, female Bengal cat presents on emergency for respiratory distress. Thoracocentesis revealed a large amount of thick brown fluid. Microscopic evaluation findings were consistent with pyothorax. A CT was performed and a cross-sectional image is shown (2).
i. In what ways can infectious agents gain access to the pleural space causing pyothorax in dogs and cats?
ii. When is surgical intervention recommended to manage pyothorax?

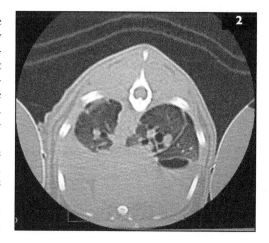

Answers: 1, 2

1i. This dog has had previous pelvic fractures resulting in a narrowed pelvic canal. The fetus did not pass through the canal and resulted in fetal death. The dog has fetal obstruction and secondary uterine inertia. Strong contractions for over 30 minutes without expulsion of a fetus indicates dystocia.

ii. A Cesarean section is recommended for the remaining living pup and for removal of the deceased trapped pup.

iii. Many anesthetic protocols have been recommended for use during Cesarean section. Puppy mortality rate is reportedly lower when propofol and isoflurane are used. Regional anesthesia has been described as an alternative to general anesthesia. The use of regional anesthesia is not correlated with improved puppy survival. Therefore, a safe protocol for Cesarean section includes induction with IV propofol without premedication, rapid intubation and maintenance of anesthesia at the lightest anesthetic plane possible. Because the fetal heart rate is low, atropine is administered. Atropine is chosen over glycopyrrolate because glycopyrrolate will not cross the placental barrier due to its large molecular weight and charge. Atropine can cause fetal disorientation or excitement due to its central action, but fetal effects may vary depending on the amount of drug absorbed.

2i. Microbial access to the pleural space is gained through penetrating injuries to the thoracic wall (bites, foreign bodies), airways (inhaled migrating plant material), esophagus or iatrogenic (thoracocentesis). Pyothorax may also be caused through hematogenous or lymphatic spread of infectious agents, pulmonary or intrathoracic neoplasia or abscessation. In rare cases, pyothorax has been identified as an extension of diskospondylitis or bronchopneumonia. It is important to note the route of infection is usually not identified in 86–96% of dogs and 33–60% of cats.

ii. Surgery by means of a lateral thoracotomy or median sternotomy is indicated when there is identification of a primary cause that requires surgical resection, such as foreign body, lung lobe torsion and/or a pulmonary abscess. Surgical intervention is also recommended when failure of appropriate medical management, which consists of systemic antimicrobial therapy and intermittent thoracocentesis or bilateral thoracostomy tube aspiration and/or lavage, occurs. Persistence of effusion beyond 3–7 days and complications associated with a previously placed thoracostomy tube are also instances when surgery is indicated. The presence of *Actinomyces* species has also been reported as an indication for surgical intervention, due to its high correlation with migrating grass awns. One paper reports short-term survival rates of 29%, 77% and 92% following treatment with thoracocentesis alone, thoracostomy tube, or thoracotomy and thoracostomy tube, respectively. In the same report, long-term survival rates for the same three groups were 29%, 71% and 70% (Boothe, 2010).

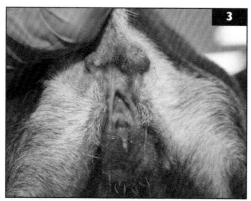

3 A 4-month-old female, mixed breed dog presents for a check-up and vaccination. The puppy has been urinating and defecating without difficulty. This is the perineum (3).
i. What is your diagnosis?
ii. What may develop as sequelae to this abnormality?
iii. What treatment is recommended?

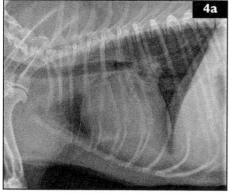

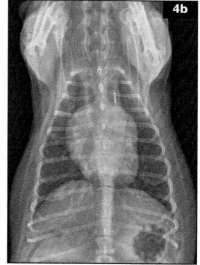

4 A 9-year-old spayed, female Shih Tzu presents for hindlimb lameness due to luxating patellas. Thoracic radiographs are shown (4a, b). A grade IV/VI left apical systolic murmur is ausculted.
i. What is the most likely cause of the murmur in this dog?
ii. Discuss special considerations for sedation and anesthesia of this patient.
iii. What would be a contraindication for surgery?

3i. This is an anogenital cleft and imperforate anus. In animals with anogenital clefts, the feces and urine enter a common cavity prior to exiting the body. In this dog, the ventral mucosa of the anus is continuous with the dorsal mucosa of the vagina – forming the cleft. The anal sac orifices can be seen dorsal to the anal opening. The dog also has an abnormally formed tail.

ii. Urination and defecation occur without difficulty. However, fecal incontinence, perineal soiling and irritation may occur. Because of the common vestibule shared by feces and urine, ascending urinary tract infections may occur and may lead to pyelonephritis.

iii. Re-forming the anus ventrally and then closing the soft tissues between the anus and vulva can repair an anogenital cleft.

4i. The most likely cause of the murmur is mitral regurgitation secondary to degenerative valve disease. This is the most common acquired heart disease in dogs and is very common particularly in older, small breed dogs. The radiograph shows that the dog has left atrial and left ventricular enlargement, which occurs with volume overload due to mitral regurgitation.

ii. The goals when dealing with a patient with mitral regurgitation are to avoid increases in afterload and preload, maintain contractility, avoid bradycardia and minimize myocardial oxygen demand. Alpha-2-agonists, such as dexmedetomidine, are potent vasoconstrictors that can significantly increase afterload and therefore are contraindicated in these cases. Instead, opioids which have minimal cardiovascular effects and low doses of acepromazine can be used. The vasodilatory effect of acepromazine can decrease afterload and actually be beneficial for mitral regurgitation. For induction, propofol and etomidate have minimal negative effects on the cardiovascular system. While ketamine can be used in cases of mitral regurgitation, it must be used carefully as it can cause vasoconstriction as a result of sympathetic stimulation. Although inhalants for maintenance of anesthesia are cardiovascular depressants, these effects can be minimized with a balanced anesthetic protocol. Should bradycardia develop with sedation or anesthesia, anticholinergics, such as atropine or glycopyrrolate, should be given. Additionally, high rates of parenteral fluid administration and fluid boluses should be avoided and careful monitoring of the respiratory rate before, during and following the procedure is important. Positive inotropes with minimal alpha-receptor activity, such as dobutamine, may be useful to maintain blood pressure and tissue perfusion if necessary.

iii. Untreated congestive heart failure is a contraindication for surgery. Cases of moderate to severe mitral regurgitation without congestive heart failure, such as the dog shown in the radiographs, are higher risk anesthetic candidates, but can often be successfully anesthetized with careful selection of anesthetic drugs.

5 A 7-year-old castrated, male domestic short hair cat presents for severe facial pruritus. The owners had recently adopted the cat as a stray that was found on their front porch. The cat was indoor/outdoor and frequently roamed the neighborhood unsupervised. They noticed that for the few days prior to presentation, the cat had been shaking his head frequently and would often scratch at the neck. On physical examination, severe facial excoriation is present along with a unilateral swelling of the left pinna (5). You suspect the cat has an aural hematoma.

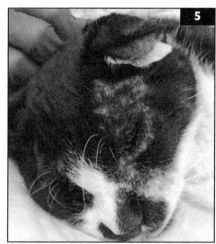

i. What additional diagnostic should be performed along with treatment of the aural hematoma?
ii. Several surgical corrections are available for aural hematomas. Describe them.
iii. The owners have moderate financial concerns and surgery is not an option for the cat. What alternative options may be considered?

6 A radiograph of an 8-year-old Labrador Retriever is shown (6). The dog presented for lameness. You plan to perform a biopsy.
i. What additional diagnostics should be performed?
ii. From where in the bone will you take the biopsy?
iii. What is a major risk of the procedure?
iv. Samples should be obtained for what other tests?

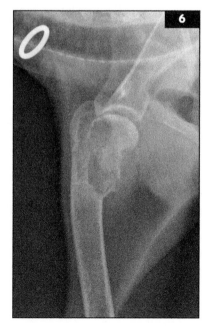

5i. Ear swabs should be collected for cytologic evaluation and to determine whether ear mites (*Otodectes cynotis*) may be a complicating factor. Aural hematomas are almost always caused by uncontrolled otitis externa. Ear mites would be a likely diagnosis in an indoor/outdoor cat; however, other options may be considered such as secondary infections (with bacteria and/or yeast), underlying allergic disease or concurrent external parasite infestation (e.g. fleas, *Notoedres* mites).

ii. Surgical techniques involve incising over the hematoma cavity, draining excess hemorrhage and placing full thickness sutures at regular intervals to keep tissue layers apposed. This tends to provide the most cosmetic repair. Alternatively, a cannula may be placed in the hematoma cavity to provide drainage. Suction drains may provide similar benefits. The cannula or drain is typically left in place for several days until drainage stops. Punch biopsy technique involves making multiple drainage holes in the pinna; the biopsy sites should be left open to heal by second intention. A CO_2 laser may be used in similar fashion to punch biopsy; tissue adherence may be improved when the laser is used.

iii. Medical treatment for aural hematomas is successful for many patients. The hematoma should be drained as much as possible (both medial and lateral compartments of the pinna may be affected) and then a small amount (approximately 0.1 mL) long-acting injectable steroid (e.g. triamcinolone acetonide) can be injected into each compartment. Bandaging may not be necessary or effective. Additionally, it is imperative to treat the inciting cause of otitis externa and any secondary infections which led to hematoma formation.

6i. In addition to the limb radiographs, three view thoracic radiographs should be performed to assess the lungs for metastatic disease. Alternatively, a thoracic CT scan could be performed. The CT scan has a greater ability to detect metastatic disease than thoracic radiographs, particularly in large breed dogs (Armbrust, 2012).

ii. The biopsy site should be chosen based on the radiographic lesion. The site should be the middle of the bony lesion. Bone biopsies are taken from the center of the bony lesion as opposed to soft tissue biopsies, which are often taken from the junction of normal and abnormal tissue. Bone biopsies are taken from a central location in order to avoid the reactive bone that surrounds the lesion.

iii. The major risk of the procedure is fracture. Fracture may occur at the time of biopsy. For that reason, radiographs should be taken following the biopsy procedure. These radiographs also help ensure that the biopsy site was appropriate. In addition to fracture at the time of biopsy, the biopsy can predispose the bone to pathologic fracture days to weeks following the biopsy procedure. Owners should be warned of this risk.

iv. In addition to histopathology, cultures may be obtained. Differentials for lytic bone lesions often include bacterial and fungal disease.

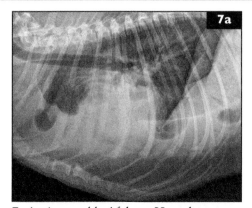

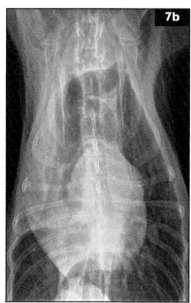

7 A 4-year-old Afghan Hound presents for increased respiratory rate and effort of several hours duration. On auscultation, the bronchovesicular lung sounds are decreased. Radiographs are made (7a, b). You suspect lung lobe torsion.

i. Which are the most commonly affected lung lobes?

ii. What are the typical changes seen on radiographs associated with lung lobe torsion?

iii. What is the prognosis following lung lobectomy in affected animals?

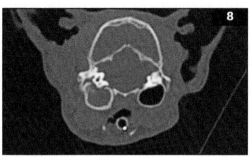

8 A 1-year-old castrated, male domestic short hair cat presents for evaluation of recurrent right ear infections and a drooping right eye. A CT scan of the head was performed (8).

i. What is your primary differential diagnosis?

ii. How can this condition be treated?

iii. How successful are the methods of treatment?

7i. Lung lobe torsion typically affects the right middle lung lobe. Nearly any lung lobe can become torsed, but the right middle and left cranial lung lobe are reported most frequently. In Pugs, the left cranial lung lobe is most commonly affected and is thought to be spontaneous in this breed, typically occurring in animals 4.5 years old or younger. A predominately male distribution is observed. Lung lobe torsion can be spontaneous or occur secondary to other intrathoracic disease, such as chylothorax. Large dogs with deep, narrow chest cavities, like the Afghan Hound, have a higher incidence of lung lobe torsion.

ii. Abnormalities associated with lung lobe torsion that can be seen on radiographs include pleural effusion and lung lobe consolidation. If the condition is detected early, an alveolar lung pattern may be observed. However, air is absorbed and replaced by fluid within 2–3 days, causing an increased fluid opacity in the lung lobe with 97% of affected lobes appearing emphysematous. The involved bronchus appears narrowed or blunted in the majority of cases. Occasionally, dorsal tracheal displacement and mediastinal shift are observed.

iii. Reported prognosis following lung lobectomy varies between studies but is thought to be more favorable in Pugs. One study reported a survival rate of 50% (Neath, 2000), while another yielded an overall survival of 61%, with 6 of 7 Pugs having a good outcome (Murphy, 2006).

8i. An inflammatory polyp is the primary differential diagnosis. Inflammatory polyps are common in young cats. The inflammatory polyps often originate in the middle ear near the junction of the auditory tube and the tympanic bulla. They may migrate into the horizontal ear canal or into the nasopharynx. The etiology of inflammatory polyps is unknown but may have a congenital origin or result secondary to middle ear disease.

ii. Inflammatory polyps are treated with traction and avulsion of the polyp from the horizontal ear canal, or an oral approach. Alternatively, ventral bulla osteotomy can be performed. The oral approach may require incision of the soft palate to gain access to the polyp.

iii. Success rates of traction and avulsion of the polyp vary based on location of the polyp. Traction and avulsion combined with orally administered prednisolone results in recurrence in only 10% of cats with nasopharyngeal polyps. Cats with external ear polyps had a 50% recurrence rate with the same treatment. Following ventral bulla osteotomy and curettage of the bulla, a recurrence rate of 2% is expected (Anderson, 2000).

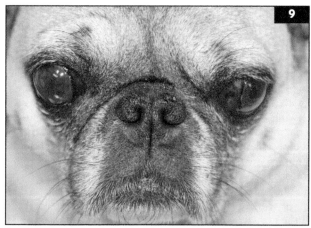

9 A 6-month-old Pug presents for an ovariohysterectomy. You examine the dog and find that the nares are stenotic (9).
i. What different surgical techniques can be performed for correction of stenotic nares? Describe each technique.
ii. What additional anatomy will you check while you anesthetize the dog for the surgical procedure?

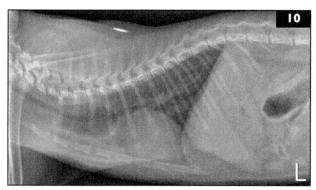

10 A 4-month-old male domestic short hair cat presents for a history of regurgitation. The regurgitation began when the cat was weaned off milk and started on food. A left lateral thoracic radiograph is shown (10).
i. Describe the radiographic findings, and tentative diagnosis.
ii. Name the subtypes of your tentative diagnosis.
iii. What imaging technique could be performed to further define the tentative diagnosis?
iv. What other differential diagnosis should be considered?

9i. Stenotic nares can be treated with vertical wedge resection, horizontal wedge resection, alapexy (Ellison, 2004), nares amputation (also known as Trader's technique) (Huck, 2008) or punch resection alaplasty (Trostel, 2010). Vertical wedge resection is performed by removing a wedge of tissue from the wing of the nostril, including a pyramid of tissue caudally in the alar cartilage. The base of the wedge is the free edge of the wing of the nostril. The horizontal wedge resection is performed with a medial to lateral oriented wedge. The mucosa on the ventral surface of the wing of the nostril is preserved and a wedge of tissue is removed just dorsal to the mucosal border. The second incision is made horizontally across the wing of the nostril and the two incisions meet at the alar fold. The incisions for both techniques are made with a #11 Bard-Parker blade and closed with interrupted, absorbable 4-0 suture material.

Alapexy is performed by making two elliptical incisions, the first on the ventrolateral skin (lateral to the wing of the nostril) and the second incision on the lateral aspect of the wing of the nostril. The edges of the incisions are apposed and sutured.

Nares amputation is performed with a single incision per side. The ventral aspect of the wing of the nostril is removed. No sutures are placed. Punch resection alaplasty is performed using a circular dermatological punch tool. A circular piece of tissue is removed from the wing of the nostril bordered laterally at the alar fold. The circular defect is sutured with interrupted sutures.

ii. Because this is a brachycephalic breed, a laryngeal exam should also be performed. This includes examination of the soft palate, larynx and laryngeal saccules.

10i. There is a gas- and fluid-dilated cranial thoracic esophagus that terminates at the level of the heart base and is causing widening of the cranial mediastinum. The trachea is deviated ventrally and to the left. These findings are consistent with a vascular ring anomaly.

ii. The most common vascular ring anomaly in dogs and cats is a persistent right aortic arch with a left ligamentum arteriosum. In this anomaly, the aortic arch develops on the right side of the animal and the ligamentum arteriosum forms in the usual location between the anomalous right aortic arch and the pulmonary artery. This combination traps the esophagus between the ligamentum arteriosum and aorta resulting in constriction of the esophagus. Other differentials occur less commonly and include aberrant right subclavian, persistent right ductus arteriosus, aberrant left subclavian, aberrant left subclavian with persistent right aortic arch and double aortic arch. Unlike the other differentials, the double aortic arch can lead to compression of the trachea and respiratory difficulty.

iii. Different imaging techniques that could be useful include barium esophagram, esophagoscopy, fluoroscopic examination of esophageal motility and contrast CT. In this case, contrast CT was subsequently performed and the vascular ring anomaly was diagnosed as an aberrant right subclavian artery.

iv. Esophageal stricture, segmental myasthenia gravis and congenital megaesophagus should all be considered.

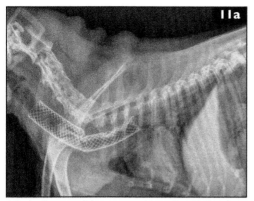

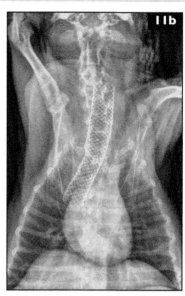

11 A 5-year-old castrated, male Chihuahua presents for difficulty breathing and a worsening cough with activity. Six months prior, a nitinol endotracheal stent was placed for treatment of a grade IV tracheal collapse. On physical examination, a mild cough is present. Radiography is performed (**11a, b**).
i. What is your diagnosis?
ii. How common is this complication? When does this complication usually occur?
iii. What surgical treatment options are available for this dog?
iv. What medical treatment options are available?

12 A fine needle aspirate from a lytic lesion in the seventh lumbar vertebra of a 6-year-old spayed, female German Shepherd dog is shown (**12**). The dog is febrile and exhibits pain on palpation of the spine.
i. What is your diagnosis based on the cytologic image?
ii. What are the two most common species of organism isolated?

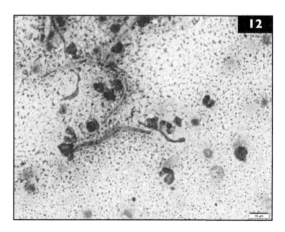

Answers: 11, 12

11i. A fracture of the tracheal stent is present at the caudal end (intrathoracic) portion of the trachea.

ii. Stent fracture is a common complication. In one report, five of 12 stents fractured within the first 6 months of placement (Sura, 2008). The stent most commonly fractures at the thoracic inlet. Once fracture occurs, it can propagate cranially and/or caudally.

iii. One surgical option for this patient is placement of a second nitinol stent telescoped inside of the first (fractured) stent. One report (Ouellet, 2006) describes resolution of clinical signs after placement of a second stent inside a fractured stent. Resection and anastomosis of the fractured stent and associated tracheal segments has also been reported (Mittleman, 2004). Tracheotomy with stent removal can also be performed. Surgical revision by placing extraluminal tracheal rings may help support the trachea after stent removal (Sura 2008). Tracheal ring placement without revision or removal of the stent is also possible; however, this would only be an option for the extrathoracic tracheal segment.

iv. Some patients do not require surgical revision and can be treated medically for tracheal collapse. Medications commonly used for tracheal collapse include tranquilizers (such as acepromazine) as needed during episodes of excitement. Cough suppressants (such as hydrocodone or butorphanol) and bronchodilators (such as theophylline) can also be helpful in some cases. Finally, short-term corticosteroids (such as prednisone) can be utilized in the acute phase and can help with inflammation and edema in the tracheal lumen. A course of antibiotics can be instituted if a secondary infection is suspected.

12i. Fungal osteomyelitis is the most likely differential. The image shows several fungal hyphal structures that are septate, and exhibit approximately 90-degree branching. The cytologic appearance of these hyphae is most consistent with *Aspergillus* species although *Penicillium* can look similarly and would also be a differential. An inflammatory cell population, consisting of macrophages and mildly to moderately degenerate neutrophils, is also seen.

ii. The two most common isolates responsible for systemic aspergillosis are *Aspergillus terreus* and *A. deflectus* (Schultz 2008). Females and German Shepherd dogs are over-represented. The most common clinicopathologic abnormalities in affected animals include leukocytosis and hyperglobulinemia (Schultz 2008). *Aspergillus* species are found in the environment and act as opportunistic pathogens. They are readily identified on cytologic or histologic examination of infected tissues.

13 A 3-year-old spayed, female domestic short hair cat presents to your hospital for wound management after being hit by a car yesterday afternoon. After thoroughly clipping and cleaning the wound, you elect to apply a honey dressing because of its many beneficial properties.
i. Describe the antimicrobial properties of honey.
ii. Describe how honey can contribute to overall tissue health and repair.

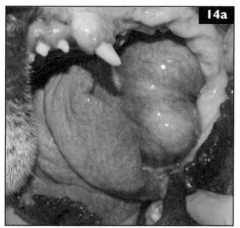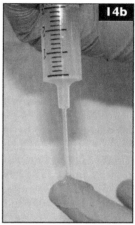

14 A 3-year-old neutered, male English Bulldog presents for evaluation of a swelling under the tongue (**14a**). Clear, blood tinged, viscous fluid was aspirated from the swelling (**14b**).
i. What is your diagnosis?
ii. What surgical procedures can be recommended?

13i. The antibacterial properties of honey have been attributed to its high osmolarity, acidity and hydrogen peroxide activity. Honey produces a low, yet therapeutic level of hydrogen peroxide, which has been shown to be effective against bacteria when continuously generated. The presence of phytochemicals within honey have been shown to be antibacterial; however, the underlying mechanism is not completely understood.

ii. The presence of high levels of natural antioxidants protects wound tissues from oxygen radicals, which may be produced by hydrogen peroxide. This may seem counterintuitive due to the above-mentioned antimicrobial effects of hydrogen peroxide; however, it is important to remember that the low levels of this agent tend to be effective against microbes. Additionally, low levels of hydrogen peroxide stimulate angiogenesis and the growth of fibroblasts. Honey contains a wide range of amino acids, vitamins and trace elements, in addition to readily assimilable sugars that stimulate tissue growth. Honey increases collagen content, accelerates collagen maturation resulting from cross-linking and maintains optimal pH conditions for fibroblast activity. Honey also provides a protective layer of protein over the wound and healthy granulation tissue.

14i. This dog appears to have a sublingual sialocele (also known as ranula). This is a collection of saliva in the subcutaneous tissue. The resultant cavity is lined by granulation tissue and the fluid aspirated from the sialocele is often viscous and clear to blood tinged. The most common cause for a sialocele is leakage of saliva from the sublingual salivary gland, but any of the salivary glands can develop a sialocele. Trauma, foreign bodies, neoplasia and sialoliths have been implicated in the development of sialoceles, but in most cases a cause is not found.

ii. Dogs with a ranula should have marsupialization of the ranula and removal of the mandibular and sublingual (both monostomatic and polystomatic) salivary glands. Marsupialization alone has been attempted. With marsupialization, a portion of the intraoral tissue is removed and the mucosa is sutured to the lining of the ranula (**14c**). The lining of the ranula is inflammatory tissue and it will attempt to heal, which may allow recurrence of the ranula.

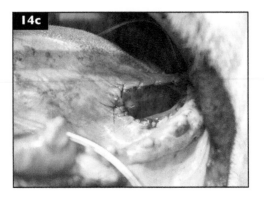

15 A 3-year-old spayed, female Bernese Mountain dog presents for evaluation of a 3-month history of polydipsia/polyuria, lethargy and recurrent urinary tract infections. Bloodwork was performed.

Analyte	Result	Reference interval
Serum total calcium	56.1 mg/dL	9.9–11.6 mg/dL
Serum phosphate	2.5 mg/dL	3–6.5 mg/dL
BUN	15 mg/dL	18–30 mg/dL
Creatinine	1.0 mg/dL	0.6–1.2 mg/dL
Serum ionized calcium	1.6 mmol/L	1.12–1.41 mmol/L
Serum parathyroid hormone	8 pmol/L	2–13 pmol/L
Serum parathyroid hormone-related protein	0.3 pmol/L	<1.5 pmol/L

i. What is the likely diagnosis?
ii. What is the most common cause of this condition?
iii. List the forms in which calcium is present in blood plasma.
iv. What controls the synthesis and release of parathyroid hormone (PTH)?
v. What are the effects of PTH and by what mechanisms do these occur?
vi. In which specific conditions may elevated parathyroid-related protein be detected?

16 A 5-year-old spayed, female Cocker Spaniel presents for recurrent ear infections. She had previously been treated medically. The owners are now unable to medicate the ears due to pain elicited during treatment. A photograph of the external ear is shown (**16**).
i. What surgical procedures can be performed for otitis externa?
ii. What surgical procedure should be recommended for this dog?

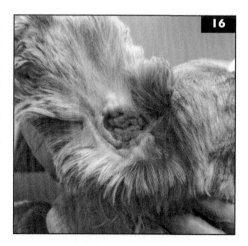

15i. Primary hyperparathyroidism.

ii. This condition is usually caused by a solitary parathyroid adenoma (90%). Less commonly, parathyroid hyperplasia (5%) and parathyroid carcinomas (5%) may occur.

iii. The majority of blood plasma calcium is present as the physiologically active ionized form (50%), with the remainder chelated to lactate, citrate and bicarbonate (10%), or protein-bound (40%).

iv. Decreasing free (ionized) calcium concentrations in blood stimulate PTH secretion by effects on calcium receptors on the chief cells of the parathyroid gland. Chief cells are responsible for synthesizing, storing and secreting PTH.

v. PTH increases serum calcium and decreases serum phosphate due to direct effects on the bone and kidney, and indirect effects on the gastrointestinal tract. Increased bone resorption occurs due to increased differentiation of macrophage precursors into osteoclasts and release of osteoclast-stimulating factors from osteoblasts. PTH directly increases the rate of calcium reabsorption at the distal convoluted tubules of the kidney and decreases the rate of phosphate absorption at the proximal tubules. PTH indirectly increases calcium absorption in the intestine through hydroxylation of vitamin D in the renal tubules.

vi. The detection of parathyroid-related protein has been associated with hypercalcemia of malignancy. Neoplasms that are commonly implicated include lymphoma and anal gland adenocarcinoma.

16i. Surgical procedures for otitis externa include: lateral wall resection, vertical canal ablation and total ear canal ablation with lateral bulla osteotomy. Lateral wall resection (Zepp procedure) is removal of the lateral portion of the vertical ear canal. This procedure increases drainage and provides ventilation to reduce moisture in the ear canal.

Vertical canal ablation is removal of the entire vertical ear canal. This procedure is used when a healthy horizontal canal is present and the vertical canal is significantly diseased. The vertical canal ablation has some benefits over lateral wall resection. These benefits include total removal of the vertical canal tissue, less postoperative exudate, less postoperative pain, and less incised cartilage resulting in better healing. Total ear canal ablation requires removal of both the vertical and the horizontal ear canals. This procedure is almost always combined with a lateral bulla osteotomy to provide access to the bulla.

ii. This dog should have a total ear canal ablation with bulla osteotomy (TECABO). TECABO is indicated in dogs with canal hyperplasia, stenosis or calcification. Additionally, it is recommended that Cocker Spaniels with recurrent otitis externa undergo TECABO.

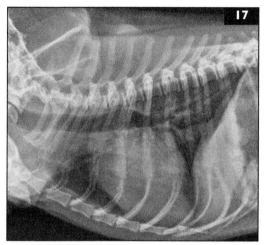

17 A 7 kg 10-year-old male Dachshund presents for removal of a subcutaneous mass from the lateral aspect of the humerus. The dog has been diagnosed with chronic valvular disease (CVD) stage C and has a past history of congestive heart failure (CHF) but is currently controlled (**17**). The dog is receiving benazepril, furosemide and pimobendan.

i. What does CVD stage C mean?

ii. What is the most appropriate anesthetic induction agent for this dog, and what side-effects can it have?

iii. What will be a suitable management of the anesthesia for this patient?

18 A photograph of a thoracocentesis being performed in a dog with chylous effusion is shown (**18**).

The cause of chylothorax in many animals is idiopathic. What are other causes of chylothorax that have been recognized in dogs and cats?

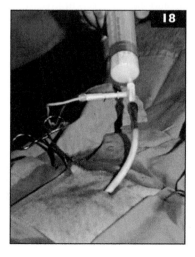

17i. CVD is the most common acquired cardiovascular disease in dogs. Four basic stages (A–D) are used to categorize pets with CVD. Stage A includes dogs at high risk to develop heart disease (Cavalier King Charles Spaniel), but that have no heart murmur. No drug or dietary therapies are recommended. Stage B includes dogs with a structural cardiac abnormality but that have never had signs of heart failure. Stage C denotes dogs with documented cardiac structural abnormality and with current or previous signs of CHF. Stage D includes patients with end-stage disease with clinical signs of heart failure that are refractory to stage C treatments (Atkins, 2009).

ii. Etomidate is an imidazole derivative anesthetic with an ultra-short action and minimal cardiac depression. Etomidate may induce excitement, myoclonus, respiratory depression and pain during injection. Also, etomidate does not abolish completely the airway reflexes and patients tend to gag and retch during intubation, making it necessary to combine it with other drugs such as benzodiazepines. Etomidate inhibits cortisol and aldosterone synthesis in the adrenal cortex for up to 6 hours after a single dose in dogs. As a result the use of etomidate may result in hyperkalemia, hyponatremia, volume depletion and reduction of systemic vascular resistance. Further, testing for Addison's or Cushing's disease should not be performed in conjunction with administration of etomidate.

iii. Goals of anesthesia are to optimize the ventricular output. This can be accomplished by minimizing the regurgitation flow and decreasing the afterload. Anesthetics, in general, tend to decrease afterload. In order to minimize the regurgitation, the heart rate should be maintained. Anticholinergics should be used conservatively since their administration may increase the myocardial oxygen consumption, compromise the myocardial perfusion and, as a result, increase the risk of ischemia. Fluids should be carefully titrated given that they can lead to pulmonary edema and pulmonary hypertension with right heart dysfunction. It is common to premedicate these animals with a low dose of an opioid, such as methadone, to avoid bradycardia. Stroke volume should be supported as needed with positive inotropes with β1 effect such as dobutamine. Balanced anesthesia utilizing a combination of fentanyl (0.8 μg/kg/min) and midazolam (8 μg/kg/min) along with low doses of isoflurane or sevoflurane will help to provide a more stable patient than if high doses of inhalants are used, since inhalants tend to depress the cardiovascular system.

18 Chylothorax can be caused by any disease or condition that increases pressure within the cranial vena cava. The increased pressure leads to obstruction of the lymphaticovenous junction, resulting in leakage of the thoracic duct/thoracic lymphatics. Conditions that can lead to increased pressure within the cranial vena cava include: masses within the mediastinum (thymoma, lymphoma), congestive heart failure, trauma, blood clot in the cranial vena cava, fungal infection, dirofilariasis and congenital anomalies. As stated above, the most common cause is idiopathic.

19 Regarding the dog in **Case 18** with chylothorax.
i. What are the typical cytologic and biochemical findings consistent with chylous effusion?
ii. List surgical options to treat idiopathic chylothorax in dogs and cats.

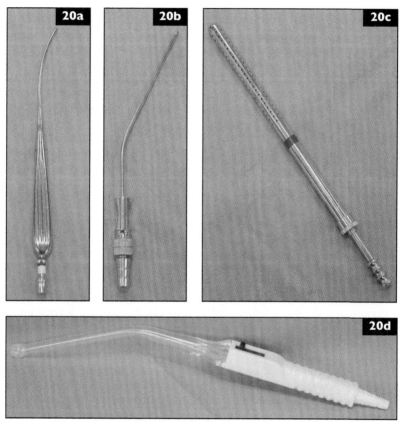

20 i. Name these surgical instruments (**20a–d**).
ii. List specific uses for each of these surgical instruments.
iii. What percentage of suction tips is contaminated during veterinary surgery and what is the likely source of contamination?

19i. Analysis of the thoracic fluid is crucial to determine if the fluid is truly chyle. The fluid is analyzed for color, clarity, type and number of cells, protein levels and the triglyceride levels. Chyle is usually classified as a modified transudate with predominantly lymphocytes. With time, non-degenerate neutrophils may become more abundant. A definitive diagnosis of chyle is made when comparing fluid triglyceride levels with serum triglyceride levels. If the triglyceride levels are higher in the fluid than in the serum, the fluid is chyle. Additionally, cholesterol levels should be measured in both fluid and serum. In chyle, cholesterol levels should be lower in the fluid than in the serum. Pseudochyle is a fluid with high cholesterol content and low triglyceride levels. Other diagnostic tests that can be performed on chylous effusion are Sudan black stain and ether clearance test. In chyle, chylomicrons are stained with Sudan black. The ether clearance test is a practical means of fluid analysis for chyle. Fluid is placed in two tubes, both tubes of pleural fluid are alkalinized and then ether is added to one tube while water is added to the other tube. Ether will dissipate the opacity while water will not – indicating a positive test for chyle.

ii. Surgical options include thoracic duct ligation, pericardiectomy, cisterna chyli ablation, omentalization, thoracic duct embolization and pleuroperitoneal or pleurovenous shunting.

20i. Cooley vascular suction tube (**20a**), Frazier suction tube (**20b**), Poole abdominal suction tube (**20c**) and Yankauer suction tube (**20d**).

ii. The Cooley vascular suction tube is designed for focused suction during vascular surgery. Its head is expanded for well-distributed suctioning across a small surface. The Frazier suction tube is indicated for pinpoint suction; an additional hole on the handle of the instrument increases the suction strength when covered. The Poole abdominal suction tube provides suction of large fluid amounts within organs and body cavities; the multiple openings reduce tissue plugging when removing fluid from cavities and the outer fenestrated portion can be removed leaving an inner pinpoint suction tube. The Yankauer suction tube also works well with removing large amounts of fluid, but the large size of the tip does not work well in delicate, small areas.

iii. The rate of contamination of suction tips during veterinary surgery is reported to be between 44% and 68%. *Staphylococcus* spp. are the predominant bacteria isolated from suction tips (Medl, 2012; Sturgeon, 2000). The source of contamination of the suction tips is suspected to be room air due to the constant inflow of air through the suction tip. However, the use of intermittent suction rather than continuous suction does not result in a lower rate of contamination of the suction tip (Medl, 2012).

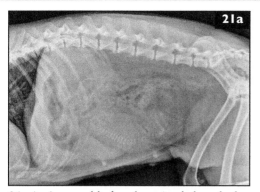

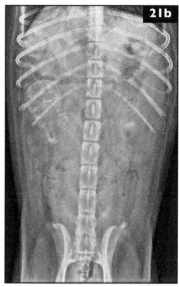

21 A 3-year-old female mixed breed dog presents for evaluation of difficulty whelping. The dog delivered three healthy pups approximately 5 hours ago. Abdominal radiographs performed 1 week prior to whelping indicated that she was pregnant with six pups (**21a, b**).
i. What are the stages of labor?
ii. What is the Ferguson reflex?
iii. What are three different surgical techniques to perform a Cesarean section?

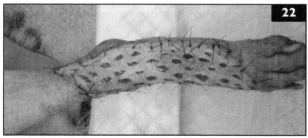

22 A dog that received a full thickness free skin graft 3 days ago presents (**22**).
i. What are the stages of free graft acceptance?
ii. What purpose(s) does meshing the graft serve?

21i. There are three stages of labor. Stage one labor includes subclinical uterine contractions and dilation of the cervix. The bitch may be restless. Respiratory rate and heart rate are usually elevated. During this time, the bitch may establish a nest. This stage of labor usually lasts 6–12 hours. During stage two labor, the puppies are expelled. The bitch has strong uterine contractions. This stage usually lasts 6–12 hours but may last up to 24 hours. Stage three labor involves expulsion of the fetal membranes and uterine involution. Fetal membranes usually pass 5–15 minutes following the birth of each pup and expulsion of pups and fetal membranes may alternate. Therefore, stage three labor can begin during stage two labor.

ii. The Ferguson reflex is a neuroendocrine reflex. A puppy moving into the birth canal or digital stimulation of the birth canal can induce uterine contractions (Ferguson reflex). Stimulation of the birth canal causes oxytocin release that enhances uterine contractions.

iii. A Cesarean section should be recommended. Surgery is initiated soon after the induction of anesthesia. Cesarean sections can be performed as an en block removal of the gravid uterus, single hysterotomy incision into the uterine body, or multiple hysterotomy incisions into the uterine horns. En bloc removal of the gravid uterus requires client approval of ovariohysterectomy prior to surgery. For en bloc removal, the ovaries are identified and their pedicles are clamped. The same is performed on the uterine body ensuring that a fetus is not close to the proposed clamp site. The entire gravid uterus is handed off to an assistant who removes the puppies. The pups should be removed from the uterus within 1 minute of clamping the uterine blood supply (Robbins, 1994).

22i. The stages of graft acceptance are adherence, plasmatic imbibition, inosculation and ingrowth of vessels. Adherence occurs early after placement of the graft. Fibrin adheres the graft to the bed. The greatest gain in strength of the fibrin occurs in the first 8 hours after application of the graft. Plasmatic imbibition is the result of capillary action of the vessels within the graft. The capillary action pulls cells and serum that have accumulated between the graft and bed into the dilated graft vessels. The absorbed fluid will diffuse into the interstitial tissues of the graft. Inosculation is the anastomosis of graft vessels with recipient bed vessels of approximately the same diameter. Inosculation may take place as early as 22 hours following placement of the graft but more frequently occurs 48–72 hours after placement. Ingrowth of new vessels occurs at a rate of approximately 0.5 mm/day. The new vessels are tortuous and dilated. The vessels mature within 48 hours and straighten and widen. The vessels continue to mature until a system of arterioles, venules and capillaries is present.

ii. Meshing the graft allows drainage, flexibility, conformity and expansion of the relocated skin.

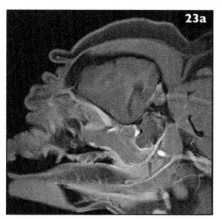
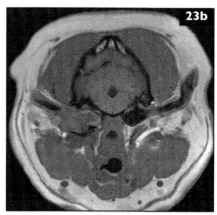

23 An 8-year-old Pug presents for what appears to be a reluctance to eat and neck pain. On examination, pain is elicited on palpation of the cranial neck. The dog also has pain on opening the mouth. An MRI of the neck and head was performed. A transverse and sagittal image is available for review (23a, b).
i. What is your diagnosis?
ii. What surgery could be performed?
iii. What is the success rate of surgery?
iv. What clinical findings have been associated with a worse prognosis?

24 An adult castrated male cat presents with a 1-day history of lethargy, abdominal discomfort and anorexia. The cat has not urinated in at least 36 hours. On physical examination, you determine that the heart rate is 60 beats per minute.
i. Describe the expected ECG abnormalities.
ii. What treatments should be administered and what is the mechanism by which the treatments work?

23i. This dog has a cholesteatoma. Cholesteatomas are lesions formed from keratinizing stratified squamous epithelium located in the middle ear. The keratinizing epithelium experiences hyperkeratosis and shedding of keratin debris. This keratin forms an expansile mass surrounded by an inflammatory reaction. Typically, interpretation of MRI images from animals with cholesteatoma reveals an expanded bulla containing material that is isointense to brain on T1-weighted images and mixed intensity on T2-weighted (Harran, 2012).

ii. Surgery should be recommended for cholesteatoma. Either a total ear canal ablation with bulla osteotomy or a ventral bulla osteotomy should be performed. Care should be given to removing all of the keratin debris and keratinizing stratified squamous epithelium.

iii. Cholesteatoma has a high recurrence rate of approximately 50%. The recurrence is likely due to keratinizing stratified squamous epithelium being left within the middle ear. Incomplete removal is likely common because the expanded bulla has an undulating appearance and removal of the lining of the bulla from all cracks and crevices is difficult (Hardie, 2008).

iv. Risk factors for recurrence of cholesteatoma after surgery are inability to open the mouth, neurologic signs on admission and lysis of the temporal bone on CT imaging (Hardie, 2008).

24i. The ECG would demonstrate a bradycardia. Additionally, the ECG tracing would be lacking P-waves and have tall, tented T-waves. All of the above findings are consistent with hyperkalemia. Occasionally, hyperkalemia will cause a tachycardia instead of bradycardia (not in this case). Hyperkalemia is most likely caused by urinary obstruction, renal failure or Addison's disease. In this cat, urinary obstruction is most likely.

ii. The cat should have several treatments concurrently. The underlying cause should be resolved appropriately. In this cat, urinary obstruction should be relieved. If the urinary bladder is enlarged and firm, the cat should have a urinary catheter placed to relieve the obstruction and allow the evacuation of urine. IV fluid therapy should be commenced with potassium deficient IV fluids. IV fluids are important to alleviate hyperkalemia by dilution and diuresis. If hyperkalemia is severe enough to cause cardiotoxicity, treatment with calcium gluconate, insulin and dextrose may be warranted. Calcium gluconate does not decrease the serum potassium levels. Instead, it raises the threshold membrane potential of the cardiac myocyte to restore cell excitability. During calcium gluconate administration, an ECG should be used to monitor the animal. Rapid administration of calcium gluconate can cause life-threatening bradycardia. Insulin and dextrose administration can be used to drive potassium into the cells and decrease serum potassium levels. During the administration of insulin, blood glucose should be monitored to recognize hypoglycemia.

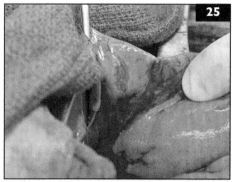

25 An intraoperative photograph from a 6-year-old German Shepherd dog is shown (25). This dog presented after increased respiratory rate and effort were noted by the owners. The dog has no known history of trauma.
i. What is your diagnosis?
ii. How can you differentiate this lesion from pulmonary cysts?
iii. What are two treatment options for this dog's condition?

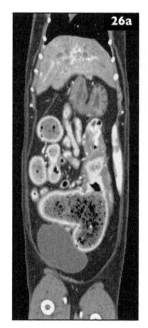

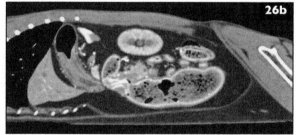

26 A 9-year-old castrated, male domestic short hair cat presents with a history of lack of appetite and decreased defecation. An abdominal ultrasound was performed that showed an intestinal mass. An abdominal CT was performed (26a, b).
i. What is your presumptive localization of the mass, based on the images provided?
ii. Name three differential diagnoses for the mass.
iii. Describe the surgical procedure, including margins.
iv. Name three surgical variations to perform this procedure.

25i. A pulmonary bulla is found within the dogs's lung. Both pulmonary bullae and blebs are air-filled blisters with fibrous walls. Bullae develop within the lung parenchyma as a confluence of alveoli. Blebs are small accumulations of air between the lung parenchyma visceral pleura that form on the surface of the lung. The air-filled spaces can be associated with obstructive diseases of the lower airways, such as blastomycosis.

ii. Pulmonary cysts can be either fluid- or air-filled and are lined by a respiratory epithelium. Cysts are most commonly seen in younger dogs and cats and are often associated with blunt thoracic trauma and pulmonary contusions.

iii. Treatment of pulmonary bullae with associated pneumothorax (if ruptured bullae) can be either conservative or surgical management. Conservative management typically involves placement of thoracostomy tubes and continuous intra-thoracic drainage. Surgical management involves a partial or complete lung lobectomy of the affected lung lobe. While improvement is seen in most patients with conservative therapy, recurrence is high. Lung lobectomy is considered the preferred treatment through a median sternotomy, as many dogs have more than one lesion or bilateral lesions. In one study of 12 dogs, no recurrence was reported after lung lobectomy for bulla or blebs (Lipscomb, 2003).

26 i. The mass appears to be arising from the orad aspect of the ascending colon.

ii. The differentials for intestinal neoplasia would include lymphoma, adeno-carcinoma, leiomyosarcoma, intestinal mast cell tumor, carcinoma, histiocytic sarcoma and liposarcoma (Bonfanti, 2006). The final diagnosis in this case was adenocarcinoma.

iii. The ideal approach would be to perform a colo-colonic anastomosis with 3–5 cm margins (to obtain wide margins around a potentially neoplastic lesion). In some cases, an ileo-colonic anastomosis is indicated if the lesion is located close to the cecum necessitating its removal. In this patient, an ileo-colonic anastomosis was performed. If the resection extends distal in the colon, near the brim of the pubis, an ileo-colonic anastomosis may be necessary as the colon is less mobile than the ileum and an ileo-colonic anastomosis may be preferred over a colo-colonic anastomosis to prevent excessive tension.

iv. Several techniques can be used for this anastomosis. Those include suture technique using simple interrupted appositional sutures, suture technique using a simple continuous suture pattern, stapling technique using a circular end-to-end anastomosis stapling device or stapling technique using gastrointestinal anastomosis (GIA) and thoracoabdominal staplers.

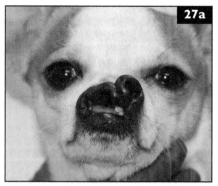
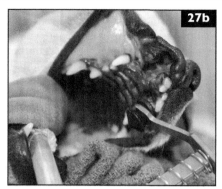

27 External (**27a**) and intraoral (**27b**) photographs of an approximately 1-year-old intact, female Chihuahua are provided. Her abnormality has been present since birth.
i. What congenital abnormality is present?
ii. What other congenital abnormalities affect the lips of dogs?
iii. What advice should be given to an owner when such an abnormality is present in their newborn puppy?

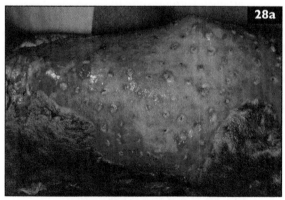

28 A surgical procedure has been performed for wound management (**28a**).
i. What procedure has been performed?
ii. Name two advantages of this type of graft.
iii. Name two disadvantages of this type of graft.

27i. This dog has a primary cleft palate. This is also known as a cleft lip or cheiloschisis. The primary palate consists of the lip and the palate rostral to the palatine fissures (alveolar process of the incisive bone). Unilateral clefts occur more frequently on the left side of the animal, although this dog has a cleft on the right side.

ii. Other congenital abnormalities affecting the lips of dogs include abnormal lip fold conformation, tight lip syndrome (Shar-Pei) and lower lip redundancy and eversion.

iii. The cleft may interfere with feeding in a newborn puppy. The owners will need to monitor the ability to nurse as some puppies are unable to latch onto the mother's nipple and suckle. If this is the case, tube feeding can be instituted to supply sufficient nutrition. Surgical closure should be attempted but should be attempted after the dog is over 8 weeks of age.

28i. This dog has had punch grafting performed. Punch grafting is a form of free graft that provides only partial coverage of the granulation bed. Punch grafts are small, full thickness skin grafts used to provide small sections of epithelialized tissue to a larger granulation bed. The epithelium from these small sections of full thickness skin advances until the entire granulation bed is covered with epithelium. The punch grafts are harvested from normal skin using a biopsy punch (6–10 mm). The harvested tissue is prepared by removing the subcutaneous tissue. Then, a 'plug' of tissue is removed from the recipient site using a smaller biopsy punch. Hemostasis is attained with pressure to the recipient site. The punch graft is then introduced into the recipient site. The area is bandaged with non-adherent bandages until the granulation bed is epithelialized. Many other types of partial coverage free grafts are described including pinch graft, strip graft and stamp graft.

ii. These grafts are easy to perform and do not require special equipment. Further, they have a high 'take' rate. Because of the uncovered granulation tissue, drainage is routinely sufficient.

iii. A major disadvantage of punch grafts is poor durability. These grafts do not cover the majority of the wound with full thickness skin. These grafts may be considered to provide a poor cosmetic appearance (**28b**).

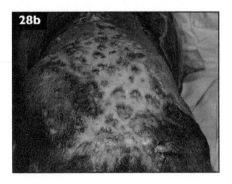

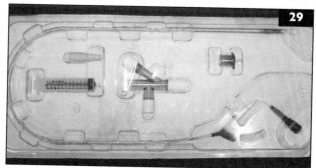

29 i. What is the device in the picture (**29**)?
ii. In what situation will it be useful?
iii. What sequelae can be expected during one lung ventilation and how can the side-effects be avoided?

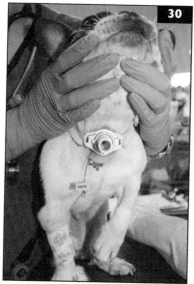

30 A French Bulldog with a temporary tracheostomy is shown (**30**).
i. What are indications for temporary tracheostomy?
ii. List three temporary tracheostomy techniques.
iii. How does one properly care for temporary tracheostomies?

Answers: 29, 30

29i. This is an Arndt endobronchial blocker utilized for lung isolation to produce one lung ventilation (OLV).

ii. The two main reasons for OLV are: (1) lung isolation, where OLV is used to protect the healthy lung from being contaminated by secretion from abscess, blood or neoplasia in the diseased lung or to redirect the ventilation away from specific areas as in cases of bullae, cysts or bronchopleural fistulae; (2) lung separation where there is no risk of contamination but improvement of the visual surgery field is needed in procedures such as pneumonectomy, thoracoscopy or cardiovascular surgery.

iii. The most remarkable changes during OLV occur in the blood gases, where arterial partial pressure of oxygen (PaO_2) tends to decrease dramatically. Pulse oxymetry (SpO_2) may reflect changes during the first minutes, but it tends to recover. However, PaO_2 does not necessarily recover, making the assessment of blood gases critical. The percentage of dead space, shunt fraction and A–a gradient (PAO_2–PaO_2; partial pressure of alveolar oxygen minus partial pressure of arterial oxygen) also increase. Moderate tidal volume (6–8 ml/kg) plus positive end expiratory pressure (up to 5 mmHg) are recommended since high volumes may increase the pulmonary resistance of the ventilated lung and potentially increase the perfusion of the non-ventilated lung, resulting in an increase in the shunting fraction (V/Q). High volumes may also impair the venous return and therefore the cardiac output. Continuous positive airway pressure (3–10 cmH_2O) may be used in the non-ventilated lung along with the administration of oxygen to prevent or to treat hypoxemia.

30i. The main indication for tracheostomy is life-threatening upper respiratory obstruction. Temporary tracheostomy may also be placed in anticipation of life-threatening upper respiratory obstruction or for surgical procedures in which access to the oral cavity, pharynx or larynx is required. If long-term support with a mechanical ventilator will be required, a temporary tracheostomy is indicated to prevent laryngeal irritation from long-term intubation.

ii. Three temporary tracheostomy techniques are: transverse tracheotomy, tracheal flap tracheotomy and vertical tracheotomy.

iii. Temporary tracheostomy care can be intense for the duration of the management time. If a cuffed tracheostomy tube has been placed, the cuff should remain uninflated unless the patient is placed on a mechanical ventilator or under general anesthesia. Regular cleaning of the tube is an important part of maintenance. Mucous production in the airways is significant. Mucous production is stimulated because the patient is breathing air that has not been humidified by the nasal passage. Tube cleaning should occur at least three times daily and more frequently in pets producing a large amount of mucous. Suctioning of the airway can be performed with a sterile suction catheter. The airway should be humidified by administering sterile saline into the tracheostomy tube every 1–4 hours.

31 The patient in **Case 30** required the creation of a permanent tracheostomy.
i. Briefly describe the procedure to create a permanent tracheostomy.
ii. What is the prognosis associated with this procedure when performed in a cat?

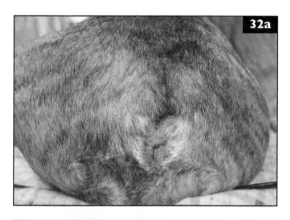

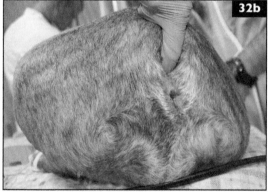

32 A 4-year-old spayed, female English Bulldog presents for evaluation of a painful, malodorous hind end with drainage coming from the tail folds. The dog scoots excessively and attempts to lick the hind end excessively. A photograph of the tail (**32a**) and of palpation of the tail bed (**32b**) are shown.
i. What is your diagnosis?
ii. What non-surgical therapy is recommended?
iii. What surgical therapy can be recommended?

31i. A permanent tracheostomy is created through a ventral midline incision. The trachea is exposed and gently dissected. The sternohyoideus muscles (right and left) are sutured together dorsal to the trachea to position the trachea nearer to the skin. The ventral half of four cartilaginous rings is excised. The tracheal mucosa is exposed and elevated slightly. The mucosa is sutured to the skin achieving perfect apposition between the mucosa and skin.

ii. The prognosis associated with permanent tracheostomy in cats is poor. In one study, cats underwent permanent tracheostomy for a variety of reasons including neoplasia, inflammatory laryngeal disease, laryngeal paralysis and trauma. Following surgery, mucous plugs leading to dyspnea were common. The median survival time of cats undergoing permanent tracheostomy was 20.5 days (range 1 day to 5 years). Cats that underwent the procedure to treat inflammatory laryngeal disease were 6.6 times as likely to die as cats that underwent the procedure for any other reason (Stepnik, 2009).

32i. This dog has tail fold intertrigo (screw tail). This condition can be found in English Bulldogs, Boston Terriers, Pugs and French Bulldogs. In more severe cases, the tail can deviate ventrally, covering the anus.

ii. The mainstay of non-surgical treatment of screw tail is cleaning the tail folds and application of topical antimicrobials. Cytologic examination of the irritated skin can be performed. Yeast and bacterial pyoderma should be treated appropriately.

iii. A caudectomy is indicated to treat this condition surgically. The caudectomy should be performed high enough to remove the deviated caudal vertebrae (**32c**).

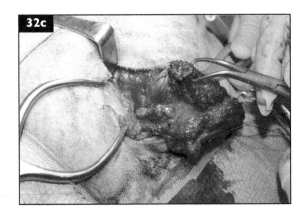

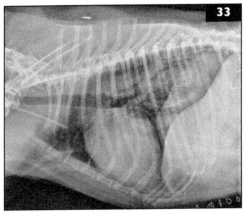

33 A 9-year-old spayed, female Jack Russell Terrier presents for evaluation of intermittent hypersalivation and regurgitation.
i. What is your diagnosis (33)?
ii. What are two types of this disorder?
iii. What breed(s) are predisposed to this disorder?

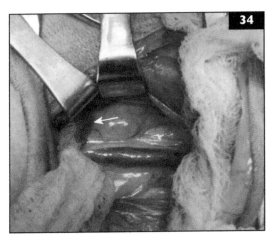

34 An intraoperative view of a cat with a tracheal avulsion is shown (34).
i. How does this injury typically occur?
ii. At what anatomic location does the trachea typically avulse?
iii. What surgical approach is used to access this location?
iv. What anatomic structure must be ligated and divided in order to access this portion of the respiratory tract (arrow)?

Answers: 33, 34

33i. This dog has a hiatal hernia. The thoracic radiographic abnormalities present in this dog are megaesophagus and a soft tissue mass dorsal to the thoracic vena cava (fundus of the stomach extending cranial to the diaphragm at the esophageal hiatus). Radiographic abnormalities that may also be associated with this condition include absence of the right crus of the diaphragmatic border and alveolar lung pattern consistent with aspiration pneumonia. This dog also has a jugular catheter in place, hemostatic clips in the abdomen and skin staples.

ii. Two types of hiatal hernia are recognized: sliding esophageal hiatal hernia and paraesophageal hiatal hernia. The most common type in dogs and cats is a sliding hiatal hernia, an axial displacement of the abdominal esophagus and a portion of the stomach through the esophageal hiatus and into the thorax. In paraesophageal hiatal hernia, the esophagogastric junction remains in place but the fundus of the stomach moves through the esophageal hiatus into the mediastinum adjacent to the esophagus. Paraesophageal hiatal hernia is rare.

iii. Shar-Pei dogs have a breed predisposition to hiatal hernia. Additionally, upper respiratory obstruction can exacerbate the clinical signs associated with hiatal hernias. Therefore, increased frequency of hiatal hernia may be seen in dogs with brachycephalic airway syndrome.

34i. This injury is considered to result from blunt trauma to the neck or thorax that involves hyperextension of the head and neck. The hyperextension stretches the trachea. Tissues that are stronger than the trachea fix the carina and lungs in position.

ii. The trachea usually ruptures intrathoracically at a position 1–4 cm cranial to the tracheal bifurcation. This is the location of the rupture because of the stronger tissues fixing the carina and lungs in position. The carina and lungs have very little 'give' and the trachea avulses from the carina.

iii. A right lateral thoracotomy at the fourth intercostal space is the approach of choice.

iv. The azygous vein is ligated and transected because it is overlying the avulsed portion of the trachea. The azygous vein must be ligated and transected for any procedure involving the dorsal mediastinum in the right side of the thorax in the cat (such as thoracic duct ligation).

35 A 7-year-old intact, male mixed breed dog presents with lethargy, straining to urinate and straining to defecate. On physical examination, a caudal abdominal mass was palpated. On rectal examination, an enlarged prostate was detected. Palpation of the prostate elicited a pain response from the dog. An abdominal ultrasound revealed an enlarged, cavitated prostate containing echogenic material. A sample of the fluid within the prostate was obtained and submitted for cytologic examination and culture (35). Cytologic examination of the fluid indicated that it was consistent with a prostatic abscess.

i. What surgical procedure(s) would you perform?
ii. What prognosis is associated with this condition?

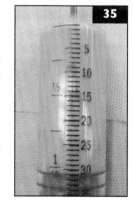

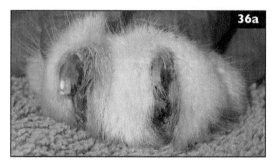

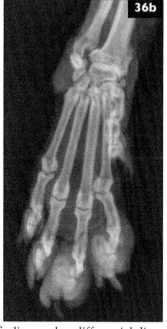

36 A 13-year-old spayed, female domestic short hair cat presents for chronic discharge around multiple claws. The owner noticed the cat limping on the left front limb approximately 4 weeks prior to presentation. Antibiotic administration failed to provide clinical resolution and the lesions continue to progress. On physical examination, purulent–hemorrhagic exudate was noted surrounding the claw fold of multiple digits on both front feet. The affected digits were severely swollen and painful on palpation (36a). Radiographs of the left front limb are shown (36b).

i. Given the clinical appearance and radiographic findings, what differential diagnoses should be considered?
ii. What additional diagnostics are recommended to help better identify the etiologic agent responsible for the lesions seen?
iii. What is 'feline lung–digit syndrome'?

35i. The surgical treatment of this dog will include castration and prostatic drainage. Castration is recommended to decrease the size and secretions of the prostate. Prostatic drainage can be achieved by many different methods including drain placement, marsupialization, omentalization and prostatectomy (partial or complete). Omentalization has been shown to provide good results. In order to omentalize the prostate, lateral stab incisions are made into the prostatic capsule. The prostate gland is palpated and a portion of the wall of the abscess is removed near the stab incisions and submitted for histopathological evaluation. Care is taken not to disrupt the prostatic urethra. The abscess is drained and lavaged generously. Omentum is packed in the prostate. If possible, the omentum is drawn through the prostatic parenchyma, dorsally to and surrounding the prostatic urethra. If the prostatic urethra is disrupted, an indwelling urinary catheter is placed for approximately 5 days.

ii. Approximately one-half of dogs with prostatic abscesses suffer from sepsis and these dogs require aggressive treatment.

36i. Bacterial paronychia, deep bacterial pyoderma (common or atypical bacterial isolates should be included on the differential list; *Staphylococcus, Mycobacteria, Nocardia, Actinomyces* species, etc.), fungal infection (opportunistic fungal infection or deep fungal mycoses including sporotrochosis, cryptococcosis, blastomycosis), immune-mediated disease (pemphigus foliaceus is most common for this location in the cat), metastatic neoplasia, foreign body reaction.

ii. Cytology of exudate, culture and susceptibility for fungal and bacterial organisms (deep tissue culture recommended), biopsy of lesions (would likely require digital amputation for adequate sample), thoracic radiographs are all recommended.

iii. 'Feline lung–digit syndrome' describes a pattern of metastatic neoplasia distinctive to cats in which a primary pulmonary neoplasm, most commonly bronchial or bronchoalveolar adenocarcinoma, metastasizes to the distal phalanges. Weight-bearing digits are most commonly affected. This uncommon condition affects older cats with no obvious sex or breed predilection. Radiographs show bony lysis of the distal phalanx with associated soft tissue swelling. Thoracic radiographs will commonly identify a solitary pulmonary nodule; however, various lung patterns have been reported. Biopsy (digit and/or pulmonary nodule) is confirmative. Prognosis is considered to be grave as no effective treatment has yet been identified for the condition (Goldfinch, 2012).

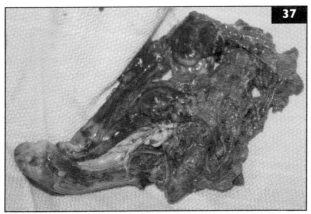

37 This adrenal mass was removed from a 10-year-old spayed, female mixed breed dog (37). The portion of the mass to the left of the photograph was removed from the caudal vena cava through a venotomy incision.

i. What is the most likely tumor type?
ii. What treatment should be administered prior to surgery?
iii. What is the prognosis associated with this surgery and disease process?

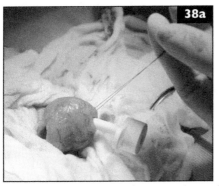
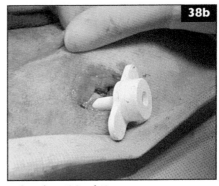

38 i. What procedure is being performed in this dog (38a, b)?
ii. List five reported indications for this procedure.
iii. What is the most common complication associated with this procedure? What is the incidence of complications associated with this procedure?

37i. Primary adrenal masses are divided into adrenocortical and medullary. Adrenocortical tumors are most likely adenomas or carcinomas. The adrenal cortex is composed of the zona glomerulosa, zona fasciculata and zona reticularis. These portions of the adrenal cortex are responsible for the production of mineralocorticoids, glucocorticoids and sex steroids, respectively. If the tumor is functional, it may induce endocrine dysfunction such as hyperadrenocorticism.

The adrenal medulla is responsible for the production of catecholamines. Adrenal medullary tumors are most likely pheochromocytomas, which originate from adrenal medullary chromaffin cells. Masses invading the caudal vena cava are most likely pheochromocytomas. The mass pictured here is most likely a pheochromocytoma because it had extensive vascular invasion. Pheochromocytomas have a prevalence of vascular invasion of 15–55% while the invasion rate for adrenocortical carcinomas is 11–21.5% (Barrera, 2013).

ii. Preoperative administration of phenoxybenzamine has been shown to improve the prognosis associated with adrenalectomy for pheochromocytoma. Phenoxybenzamine is an alpha-adrenergic antagonist that irreversibly binds to both alpha-1 and alpha-2 adrenergic receptors and blocks the alpha-adrenergic response to epinephrine and norepinephrine. This inhibition may provide a more stable patient during the perioperative period.

iii. Overall, a 20% mortality rate is associated with adrenalectomy. Mortality rates were improved by the preoperative administration of phenoxybenzamine (13% vs. 48%) (Herrera, 2008). Extension of the tumor thrombus also determines prognosis. Dogs that have caval tumor thrombi extending cranial to the hepatic hilus are four times more likely to die during the postoperative period as dogs that have thrombi that do not extend past the hepatic hilus (Barrera, 2013).

38i. This dog has a cystostomy tube. In this example, a low profile tube is being used.

ii. Detrusor atony (neurologic or idiopathic), urinary tract rupture (traumatic or iatrogenic), obstructive urinary tract neoplasia, urinary diversion following urogenital surgery, obstructive urolithiasis, feline lower urinary tract disease.

iii. A 49% complication rate is reported in dogs and cats with cystostomy tubes. The most common complication is inadvertent tube removal (Beck, 2007).

39 This dog underwent a total ear canal ablation with bulla osteotomy (TECABO).
i. What complication is this dog exhibiting?
ii. What other complications are commonly associated with TECABO? With what prevalence do these complications occur?

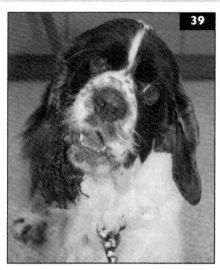

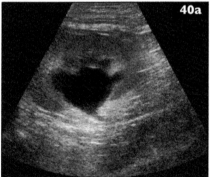

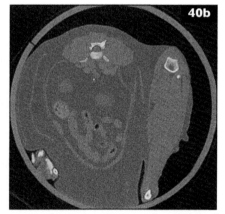

40 A 10-year-old neutered male cat presents with vomiting, lethargy and anorexia. A serum biochemistry profile was performed and showed a BUN of 45 mg/dl (reference range 19–33 mg/dL) and creatinine of 3.3 mg/dl (reference range 0.8–1.8 mg/dL). An abdominal ultrasound was performed and found hydronephrosis of the right kidney (40a) and a small, irregular left kidney. An abdominal CT examination was performed without the administration of contrast (40b).
i. What is your diagnosis?
ii. Describe the findings on the CT.
iii. What surgical procedure can be performed?
iv. What prognosis will you give this cat following ureterotomy?

39i. This dog has a head tilt associated with vestibular abnormalities. Head tilt following TECABO is a relatively uncommon complication, reported in 11% of animals undergoing TECABO. Some animals with head tilt will also have nystagmus (4.5% of animals undergoing TECABO). In most animals, head tilt is temporary and resolves within 2 months (Spivack, 2013). When this dog is examined, a palpebral response cannot be elicited indicating facial nerve paralysis is also present.

ii. Nerve damage is a common complication associated with TECABO. The facial nerve courses ventral to the ear canal and is susceptible to damage during dissection. Postoperative facial nerve deficits are reported in 48.9% of animals undergoing TECABO. Approximately one-half of the deficits are permanent while the other half resolve in 2–4 weeks (Spivack, 2013). Treatment administered to animals with facial nerve paralysis includes lubrication to the ipsilateral eye.

Facial nerve paralysis prevents blinking and distribution of the tear film. Therefore, artificial tears are often required. If indicated, fluorescein stain should be administered to the eye to monitor for corneal ulcers. If found, corneal ulcers should be treated. Horner's syndrome can result from damage to the sympathetic fibers running through the middle ear. Overall, Horner's syndrome is diagnosed in 8.2% of animals following TECABO. This complication is much more commonly elicited in cats than in dogs (3.3% of dogs following TECABO, 58.3% of cats following TECABO). Incisional complications including surgical site infection and development of draining tracts are also reported. Minor incisional complications occur in approximately 5% of animals undergoing TECABO. Draining tracts may develop as a result of incomplete removal of epithelium lining the bulla. This is an uncommon complication that can occur months to years following TECABO surgery.

40i. This cat has a right sided ureterolith.

ii. A mineral opacity is present in the right ureter. There is dilation of the ureter proximal to the mineral opacity.

iii. Depending on the location of the stone and condition of the ureter, a ureterotomy, ureteral resection and reimplantation (neoureterocystostomy), ureteral anastomosis (ureteroureterostomy or transureteroureterostomy) or ureteral replacement can be performed.

In some cases, a nephroureterectomy can be performed. This cat had a small, irregular left kidney. In order to determine if the left kidney is functioning and the right kidney is safe to remove, a renal scintigraphy (glomerular filtration rate) should be performed prior to nephroureterectomy. Ureteral stenting is an additional surgical option. Ureteral stenting is a surgical procedure in most cats, but in large dogs it can be performed minimally invasively with the aid of cystoscopy and fluoroscopy. In cats and small dogs, ureteral stenting can be performed as a 'hybrid' procedure where both surgery and fluoroscopic guidance are utilized.

iv. Cats undergoing ureterotomy have been reported to have an approximately 20% mortality rate. Uroabdomen occurs in approximately 16% of cats undergoing ureterotomy. Once cats survive 1 month postoperatively, their prognosis is good with a 1-year survival rate of 91% (Kyles, 2005).

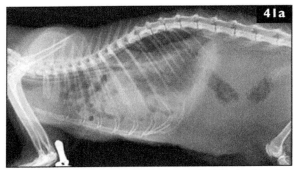

41 A lateral thoracic and abdominal radiograph (41a) of a 9-year-old spayed, female domestic short hair cat with an acute onset of labored breathing is shown. The cat is an indoor/outdoor cat.

i. Describe the radiographic findings and provide a diagnosis.

ii. What other imaging methods could be performed to provide a conclusive diagnosis?

iii. When is rapid surgical intervention of this condition required?

iv. What are potential complications of surgical intervention?

42 An arterial blood gas is taken from a 10-year-old, 50 kg female Golden Retriever undergoing an exploratory laparotomy for resection of a mass found in the small intestine. The dog has a body condition 8/9 and history of diarrhea. The anesthetic protocol included premedication with methadone and induction with propofol. The dog is being maintained under anesthesia with isoflurane delivered in 100% (FiO2) oxygen, using a rebreathing circuit with a Tec 3 vaporizer and a fresh oxygen flow of 6 ml/kg/min and breathing spontaneously. The blood sample is taken at the beginning of surgery because there are difficulties keeping the animal in a good plane of anesthesia.

pH	7.10	Cl^-	124 mEq/L
PaO_2	120 mmHg	K^+	3.8 mEq/L
SaO_2	99.9%	Lactate	1.8 mmol/L
PCO_2	47 mmHg	HTC	38%
HCO_3^-	9.8 mEq/L	TP	6.5
Na^+	143 mEq/L	Base excess	-18 mEq/L

i. Define the acid–base status of this patient.

ii. Analyse the PaO_2.

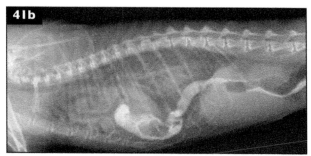

41i. Gas-filled viscera are present within the thoracic cavity. There is loss of the normal diaphragmatic line. In addition, the cardiac silhouette is obscured and few abdominal organs can be seen within the abdomen. These findings indicate diaphragmatic hernia, likely of traumatic origin.

ii. Positional radiography, administration of gastrointestinal contrast (**41b**), thoracic/abdominal ultrasonography or pneumoperitonography can be performed to provide a conclusive diagnosis. Here, contrast was administered per rectum.

iii. Immediate intervention is indicated when the stomach is herniated into the thorax. Dilation of the herniated stomach can cause rapid respiratory compromise. Additionally, the presence of non-viable bowel and a large volume of herniated abdominal organs that prevents pulmonary expansion are indications for immediate surgery.

iv. Complications include re-expansion pulmonary edema, pneumothorax, hypoxemia, hypothermia, vomiting and loss of abdominal domain requiring abdominal organ (spleen) resection to allow closure of the abdomen.

42i. Normal blood gas values are: pH 7.35–7.45; PaO_2 500 mmHg on 100% O_2; HCO_3^- 22–27 mEq/L; $PaCO_2$ 35–45 mmHg. This dog's pH indicates acidemia (pH of less than 7.35). The dog has a loss of HCO_3^- indicating a metabolic acidosis. A decrease of 0.7 mmHg in PCO_2 is expected for each 1 mEq/L decrement of HCO_3^-; therefore, the PCO_2 in this patient should be between 26 and 36 mmHg, but it is 47 mmHg, indicating that this patient is undergoing hypoventilation and respiratory acidosis. Acute respiratory acidosis is expected to produce a metabolic compensation, increasing bicarbonate by 0.15 mEq/L for each 1 mmHg increase of PCO_2, meaning that 0.3–1.8 mEq/L increase in HCO_3^- would be expected in this case. Here, HCO_3^- is just 9.8 mEq/L. If this dog were ventilating to normocapnia, the bicarbonate could be even lower. Therefore, this dog presents a mixed acid–base disorder with normal anion gap.

ii. The PaO_2/FiO_2 ratio in this patient is 120 reflecting severe venous admixture representing severe oxygenation inefficiency. The typical five reasons for this increase in venous admixture are: (1) increase in the units with high ventilation and low perfusion (dead space); (2) increase in the units with low ventilation and high perfusion (shunting); (3) diffusion barrier problems; (4) low venous oxygen content; and, (5) anatomical right to left shunts.

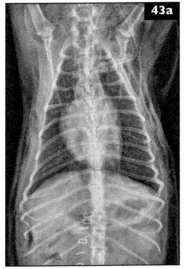
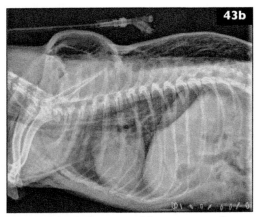

43 A 5-year-old female Shih Tzu presented for lethargy and inappetence. Severe hydronephrosis was diagnosed and a nephrectomy was performed. Under the same anesthetic, an esophageal feeding tube was placed. All procedures were performed without complication. The following morning, this radiograph was made (43a, b).
i. What are the radiographic findings?
ii. What is the most likely cause in this patient?

44 A 3-year-old spayed, 30 kg female Labrador Retriever presents for an acute onset of vomiting and inappetence. The dog has a history of dietary indiscretion. On physical examination, she is estimated to be approximately 10% dehydrated, is tachycardic (heart rate 180 bpm) and abdominal pain is noted. Abdominal radiographs are suggestive of small bowel obstruction. Bloodwork reveals hemoconcentration (PCV 58%) but is otherwise unremarkable.
i. Prepare a preoperative intravenous fluid therapy plan for this patient. Include fluid type, rate, and monitoring parameters.
ii. Prepare a postoperative intravenous fluid therapy plan for this patient. Assume that patient is euhydrated upon recovery.
iii. What are the potential risks of administering lactated Ringer's solution (LRS) to this patient postoperatively?

43i. There is severe subcutaneous emphysema in the cervical region, along the thoracic body wall and along the abdominal body wall. The cranial mediastinal structures are surrounded by free gas (pneumomediastinum). The heart is normal in size and shape. Pulmonary parenchyma is normal in opacity. An esophageal feeding tube is in place and terminates at the level of the ninth rib. There is a small volume of free peritoneal gas consistent with surgery performed the previous day. There is gas within the cervical esophagus.

ii. The likely cause of the subcutaneous emphysema and pneumomediastinum is tracheal laceration. The most likely cause of tracheal laceration is over inflation of the endotracheal tube cuff or movement of the endotracheal tube with an inflated cuff. The presence of an esophageal feeding tube is likely unrelated. The feeding tube is not placed within the airway and is appropriately positioned.

44i. The dog is dehydrated and, although surgery should not be delayed, attempts should be made to rehydrate prior to general anesthesia and surgery. The patient's fluid deficit should be calculated using: body weight (kg) × % dehydration = fluid deficit (L). If clinical signs are acute, the deficit volume can be replaced quickly. A replacement crystalloid fluid (0.9% saline, LRS, Ringer's, Normosol–R, Plasmalyte-A, Plasmalyte 148) should be selected. Replacement fluids have electrolyte concentrations that resemble extracellular fluid. In this specific case, the fluid deficit is calculated: 30 kg × 0.10 = 3 L. The total volume can be replaced rapidly (over approximately 30 minutes to 2 hours) as the dog is being prepared for surgery. To evaluate hydration status, repeat the physical examination (including mucous membrane color, capillary refill time, skin tent/turgor) and body weight can be re-evaluated. As the fluid deficit is corrected, you can expect the patient to gain 3 kg in body weight.

ii. Postoperatively, if the patient is euhydrated, maintenance IV fluids can be administered. Maintenance fluid can be calculated using: body weight (kg) × 60 mL = maintenance fluid rate (mL/kg/day). A maintenance crystalloid should be selected (0.45% saline, 2.5% dextrose in 0.45% saline, 2.5% dextrose in half strength LRS, Normosol-M, Normosol-M in 5% dextrose, Plasmalyte 56, Plasmalyte 56 in 5% dextrose). Maintenance crystalloids contain electrolyte concentrations that are meant to replace electrolytes lost daily through urine and feces. This fluid type and rate should be adequate as long as there are not any additional complications or ongoing fluid losses. In this dog, the maintenance fluid calculation is 30 kg × 60 mL = 1,800 mL/day (75 mL/h).

iii. LRS is a replacement solution and is not intended for long-term maintenance use. Short-term administration is unlikely to cause significant problems but long-term use can lead to electrolyte abnormalities (hypernatremia and hypokalemia).

45 A 7-year-old spayed, female Bulldog mix presents following a 3-day history of vomiting. Two days ago, a barium series was performed on this dog. On presentation, the dog is laterally recumbent, tachypneic and tachycardic. You perform abdominal radiographs (45a).

i. What is your diagnosis? What additional radiographic views can be performed to confirm your suspicion?

ii. What is your surgical recommendation?

iii. What prognosis do you give the owners?

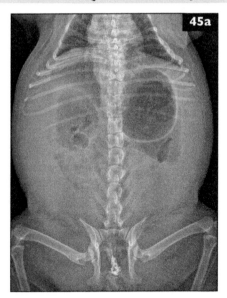

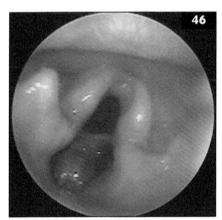

46 An endoscopic photograph, taken during laryngeal exam of a 10-year-old castrated, male Dachshund under mild sedation, is shown (46). Examination was performed because of a reported 6-month history of exercise and heat intolerance.

i. What is your diagnosis?

ii. What are the most common surgical procedures that are associated with the formation of this abnormality?

iii. What surgical interventions have been described as treatment for this condition?

45i. The radiographs of this dog show a moderate volume of free air in the abdomen and significant reduction in serosal detail. Several curvilinear ill-defined regions of mineral opacification are present within the abdomen consistent with barium within the peritoneal space. In order to confirm the presence of free air in the abdomen, a cross-table horizontal beam view may be performed while the dog is in lateral

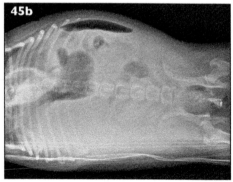

recumbency (**45b**). Given no recent history of abdominal surgery or abdominal puncture, a perforated hollow viscus is suspected. No foreign body or intestinal obstructive pattern is seen on this radiograph, although moderate gas distention of intestinal segments is present. The lack of an obstructive pattern does not rule out the possibility of an intestinal foreign body leading to perforation of the gastrointestinal tract in this case. In an older animal, a ruptured gastrointestinal tumor should be given high consideration.

ii. An abdominal exploratory surgery should be performed as soon as possible. The underlying cause should be identified and rectified and foreign material should be removed. At least 200–300 mL/kg of saline solution should be used initially to flush the peritoneal cavity. Additionally, the use of active drainage and a jejunostomy tube should be considered.

iii. The chance of survival following surgery and aggressive postoperative management is approximately 64–71% (Staatz 2002, Lanz 2001).

46i. Ventral glottic stenosis secondary to laryngeal web formation.

ii. Formation of laryngeal webbing is most commonly associated with surgery of the larynx, most commonly oral ventriculocordectomy (66.7% incidence). Other cited surgical interventions associated with laryngeal web formation include arytenoid lateralization, unilateral arytenoidectomy and bilateral laryngeal sacculectomy. Clinical signs typically begin within 1–4 months following laryngeal surgery and can include exercise intolerance, heat intolerance, stridor, dyspnea and collapse.

iii. Ventral laryngotomy with primary mucosal closure after laryngeal web resection has been reported to result in resolution of clinical signs in 67% at long-term follow-up. This approach allows for complete resection of scar tissue and primary closure of the mucosal defect. Mucosal apposition has been found to preserve airway size in experimental models of acquired laryngeal webbing. Resection of laryngeal webbing followed by oral administration of glucocorticoids or direct application of inhibitors of fibroblast proliferation has been reported. Mitomycin C and Chitosan have been experimentally shown to reduce occurrence of glottic stenosis through this inhibition after a 5-minute topical application.

47 A 12-year-old neutered, male domestic short hair cat presents for weight loss and hyperactivity. The cat was diagnosed with hyperthyroidism and management was attempted with methimazole. Unfortunately, the cat developed adverse effects to methimazole and surgical thyroidectomy was elected. A preoperative technetium scintigraphy scan was performed. The scintigraphy scan indicated

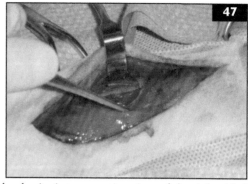

bilateral hyperfunctioning thyroid glands. An intraoperative view of the right sided surgical site following excision of both thyroid glands is shown (**47**).
i. What are the neurovascular structures that are near the surgical field and must be protected during this procedure?
ii. What are the different methods of thyroidectomy?
iii. In this case of bilateral thyroidectomy, what electrolyte must be carefully monitored postoperatively and why?

48 A 2–year-old American Pit Bull Terrier presents with pain and discomfort around the ear and hemorrhage from the ear canal after being hit by a car. An exploratory surgery through a caudal approach to the ear canal is performed (**48**).
i. What is the diagnosis?
ii. What are the treatment options for this condition?

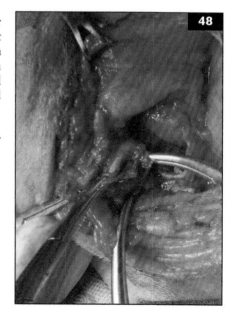

47i. The neurovascular structures near the right surgical field include the carotid artery, internal jugular vein and vagosympathetic trunk. The recurrent laryngeal nerve is also nearby, coursing dorsal to the thyroid gland and in close association with the trachea. The left thyroid gland is partially separated from the carotid sheath by the esophagus. The blood supply to the thyroid gland comes from the cranial thyroid artery. The caudal thyroid artery is present in the dog but not in the cat.

ii. Thyroidectomy has been described as intracapsular, extracapsular and modified extracapsular. In the intracapsular technique, the capsule is incised and the thyroid gland is bluntly removed from its capsule. The extracapsular technique is useful in unilateral disease. The external parathyroid gland is sharply dissected from the thyroid capsule and the entire thyroid gland is removed without penetrating the thyroid capsule. The modified extracapsular technique was developed to prevent ischemia of the parathyroid gland. In the modified extracapsular technique, the thyroid capsule is incised approximately 2 mm from and circumferentially around the parathyroid gland. The blood supply to the parathyroid gland is preserved and the parathyroid gland is dissected from the thyroid gland. The remaining thyroid gland and capsule are dissected and removed. A main benefit of the modified extracapsular technique is sustained blood supply to the parathyroid gland and reduced chance of postoperative hypocalcemia. The main drawback to the intracapsular technique is that the thyroid capsule is not removed. This increases the chance of leaving residual thyroid tissue.

iii. When bilateral thyroidectomy is performed, postoperative hypocalcemia is likely. The ionized calcium levels should be monitored and calcium gluconate should be administered if needed. Any of the techniques of thyroidectomy may lead to compromise of the parathyroid gland and resultant hypocalcemia.

48i. Traumatic separation of the auricular and annular ear cartilage.

ii. Treatment is surgical and depends on the type of ear canal separation and chronicity of the problem. Ear canal separation is divided into separation between the auricular and annular cartilage (more common) and avulsion of the annular cartilage from the acoustic meatus (uncommon). Primary repair with anastomosis of the auricular and the annular cartilage should be attempted. Total ear canal ablation and lateral bulla osteotomy may be reserved to treat failures, avulsion of the annular cartilage from the acoustic meatus or in cases of para-aural abscessation or otitis media.

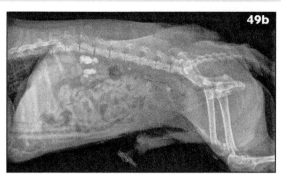

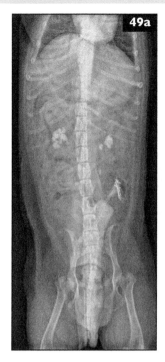

49 A 10-year-old castrated, male Shih Tzu presents for evaluation of straining to urinate. The dog has been intermittently straining for the past 3 weeks. On the day of presentation, the dog is unable to pass urine. On physical examination, the urinary bladder is firm and large. A urinary catheter is placed and the bladder is emptied. Abdominal radiographs are performed (49a, b).
i. Interpret the radiographs.
ii. What is your diagnosis?
iii. Which type of stone is the most likely in this dog?

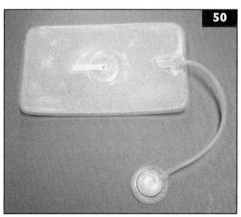

50 i. Name this surgical implant (50).
ii. How is it used?
iii. By what physiologic mechanism does it perform its intended function?

49i. Several large, mineral opacity calculi are present in each kidney and within the ureters. Two mineralized calculi are present within the intrapelvic urethra. A single, small calculus is identified within the urinary bladder. The dog has an indwelling urinary catheter which has staples associated with it at the tip of the prepuce.

ii. This dog has urinary calculi. The two calculi in the intrapelvic urethra are likely causing the urinary obstruction.

iii. In uroliths removed from the upper urinary tract (kidney and ureter), calcium oxalate stones are more common with struvite being the second most common. The stones in this dog are radiopaque, which would make both calcium oxalate and struvite possible. Calcium oxalate stones are more commonly identified in male dogs while struvite stones are more commonly identified in female dogs. Further, oxalate stones are found more frequently in older dogs, while struvite stones are found more often in younger dogs. Additionally, the Shih Tzu breed has been shown to be at a substantially higher risk of developing calcium oxalate uroliths. Because this is an older, male, Shih Tzu dog with radiopaque stones in the upper urinary tract, calcium oxalate stones are the most likely. Calcium oxalate stones cannot be dissolved using medical management and surgery is indicated to remove the stones if they are causing a problem such as urinary obstruction (Low, 2010).

50i. This is a skin expander or tissue expander. This implant consists of an inflatable silicone device that is attached to an injection port. The inflatable device is of a predetermined volume.

ii. The deflated tissue expander is implanted subcutaneously adjacent to a skin defect. The skin incision that is created to implant the tissue expander is allowed to heal for several days. After the healing period, inflation of the tissue expander is commenced. Inflation is achieved by injection of sterile saline or sterile lactated Ringer's solution into the injection port. Approximately 10% of the predetermined tissue expander volume is injected every 2 days until the final volume is achieved.

iii. The tissue expander relies on biologic creep. Biologic creep is the creation of new dermal and epidermal components after prolonged, constant loading. When using a tissue expander, the subcutaneous fat and dermal thickness decrease and the epidermis proliferates. Skeletal muscle overlying (panniculus) or underlying the tissue expander atrophies in response to increased pressure. Skin perfusion is increased because of the delay phenomenon. This occurs because blood circulation to the skin is acutely decreased when the tissue expander is placed subcutaneously. In response to the decreased blood circulation, collateral vessels respond by expanding.

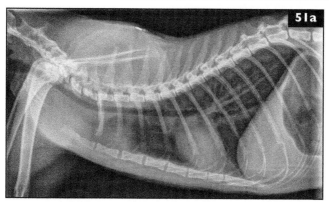

51 A 9-year-old spayed, female domestic short hair cat is admitted for inappetance, generalized weakness and cervical ventroflexion. Chest radiographs show evidence of a mediastinal mass (**51a**). Based on the clinical signs and history, you are concerned about myasthenia gravis (MG).
i. What is the best test to diagnose acquired MG definitively?
ii. What is the most likely differential for the mediastinal mass?
iii. Describe the treatment options for this patient, including both medical and surgical therapies.

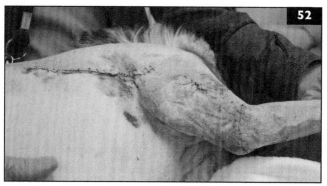

52 A photograph of a surgical wound 1 week after removal of a skin tumor is shown (**52**).

Surgical apposition of tissues with sutures or staples immediately after wound creation is considered what type of wound closure?

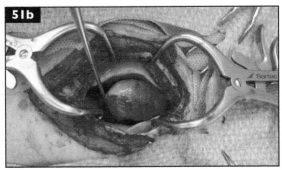

51i. MG is definitively diagnosed by identifying acetylcholine (ACh) receptor antibodies in a serum sample. Administration of edrophonium chloride (Tensilon) and seeing clinical improvement of the patient's generalized weakness can be used to support the diagnosis, but this test is reported to have a high rate of false positives and false negatives. Electrodiagnostics, such as repetitive nerve stimulation, can also be used to confirm the suspicion of MG, but other disease processes can have the same result. The gold standard remains the identification of ACh receptor antibodies.

ii. The mediastinal mass is most likely a thymoma, as they can be present in up to 25% of feline cases. MG is a common paraneoplastic syndrome associated with thymoma. Thymic monocytes in the neoplastic thymus may become immunogenic and form antibodies against ACh, resulting in MG.

iii. Surgical removal of the thymoma may be performed (**51b**), although the benefits of surgery leading to resolution of the myasthenic signs in the cat are unknown. Medical therapy is directed at increasing the availability of ACh at the neuromuscular junction through the use of anticholinesterase drugs such as neostigmine or pyridostigmine. If resolution of signs is not complete, immuno-suppression may need to be instituted in the form of high-dose prednisone, azathioprine, cyclosporine or mycophenolate mofetil.

52 With primary wound closure, or healing by first intention, the wound edges are apposed with minimal or no gap. In primary wound healing, there is minimal wound contraction, epithelialization and scar formation. Healing is rapid because the wound size is smaller. Second intention healing, or healing by contraction and epithelialization, occurs when the wound is left to heal by contraction and epithelialization. Second intention healing eventually forms a continuous epithelial surface. Third intention healing, or secondary closure, describes apposition of wound edges with suture or staples after the wound is 3–5 days old and has formed granulation tissue in the wound bed.

53 The pictured wound healing in **Case 52** is characterized by what biologic stages?

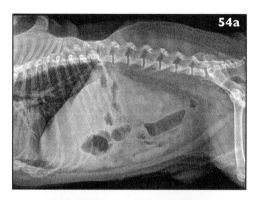

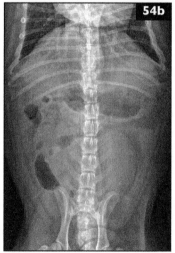

54 A 12-year-old spayed, female Toy Poodle presents with a 4-day history of vomiting, lethargy, decreased appetite and dysuria. The dog is febrile on presentation. Lab work is performed and the dog has an inflammatory leukogram and urinary tract infection. Abdominal radiographs are shown (**54a, b**).
i. Once the patient is stabilized, what is the recommended treatment?
ii. What is the likely type of finding present?
iii. What are two surgical approaches for this treatment?
iv. List advantages and disadvantages of the two techniques.
v. What is a contraindication for pyelolithotomy?

53 Primary wound closure is marked by three stages of healing: inflammation, repair and maturation. The inflammatory stage is characterized by migration of leukocytes (mainly neutrophils and monocytes) into the wound. The neutrophils remove contamination and cellular debris and are present in larger numbers early in the inflammatory phase. Later in the inflammatory phase, monocytes become the primary leukocyte and become wound macrophages. The macrophages' presence is vital for wound healing to progress. The macrophage is an important source of growth factors and mediators that modulate wound healing. The inflammatory stage typically lasts 1–3 days. The repair phase is marked by angiogenesis, fibroplasia, wound contraction and epithelialization. The transition between inflammation and repair phases is marked by the invasion of fibroblasts and accumulation of collagen in the wound. The repair phase generally lasts from days 3 to 14. The maturation phase of wound healing is the transition of the wound into a scar by remodeling of the connective tissue content of the wound. The cellularity of the granulation tissue is reduced; the collagen fiber bundles become thicker, increase in cross-linking and take on specific orientation along the lines of tension. The maturation phase can last weeks to many months.

54i. Surgical removal of the nephrolith and systemic antibiotic therapy based on culture and sensitivity is indicated. Lithotripsy has also been reported as an alternative to surgery for the management of nephrolithiasis.
ii. Calcium oxalate is the most common nephrolith.
iii. Either nephrotomy or pyelolithotomy could be performed. If the affected kidney is non-functional, a nephrectomy can be performed. If the affected kidney is infected or hydronephrotic, nephrectomy can be considered if the contralateral kidney is functioning well.
iv. Pyelolithotomy does not traumatize renal parenchyma, causes minimal hemorrhage and does not require occlusion of renal vasculature, thus minimizing potential compromise of renal function. Nephrotomy allows biopsy of kidney parenchyma concurrent with the procedure. The renal pelvis can be explored and probed during nephrotomy. Nephrotomy can be performed with either a bisectional or intersegmental technique. Debate exists as to the degree of renal dysfunction induced by these techniques, but some believe that intersegmental nephrotomy leads to less parenchymal damage to the kidney. However, no difference in glomerular filtration rate has been detected between the two techniques.
v. In order to perform a pyelolithotomy, the proximal ureter and renal pelvis must be dilated. Therefore, a normal proximal ureter and renal pelvis would be considered a contraindication.

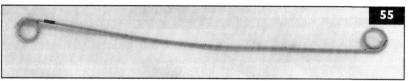

55 i. Name the device (55).
ii. Name at least five treatment options for animals with obstructive ureterolithiasis.
iii. What are the reported short- and long-term complications of ureteral stenting in dogs and cats?
iv. How can dysuria following ureteral stent placement be treated?
v. What is the reported perioperative mortality rate with ureteral stent placement and how does this compare with that of ureteral surgery?

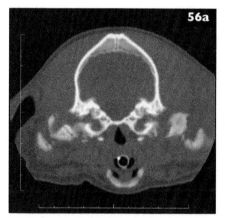
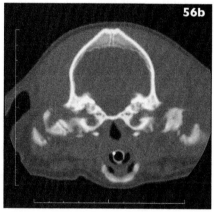

56 A 10-year-old Cocker Spaniel presents for a healing abscess below the right ear canal. The primary veterinarian had treated the abscess with local lavage and drainage as well as a course of antibiotics. A CT scan of the dog's head is performed and two consecutive images are shown (56a, b).
i. What is your diagnosis?
ii. What surgical treatment(s) would you recommend?
iii. If a mass were present within the external ear canal, what would be the most likely type?

55i. This device is a double locking-loop pigtail catheter. It is also known as a ureteral stent.

ii. Animals with obstructive ureterolithiasis can be treated by medical management, nephrostomy tube placement, dialysis, ureterotomy, ureteral reimplantation, ureteronephrectomy and ureteral stenting. Medical management consists of diuresis and attempting to allow the animal to pass the stone into the urinary bladder. During this process, aggressive fluid therapy and pain management should be instituted. Most likely, multiple imaging studies will be required in order to determine if the stone is moving. If the stone is moving, medical management can be continued. If the stone is static, the other treatment options should be considered. Nephrostomy tube placement and hemodialysis do not relieve the ureteral obstruction. Instead, each of these options can stabilize the animal until definitive treatment is attempted.

iii. The most commonly reported short-term complication reported with ureteral stenting is dysuria. Long-term complications include urinary tract infection, pollakiuria, stent migration, stent occlusion, ureteritis, tissue ingrowth, chronic hematuria and ureterovesicular reflux.

iv. Dysuria following stent placement can be treated with a short course of glucocorticoid therapy.

v. The perioperative mortality rate associated with ureteral stenting is reported to be less than 10% in both dogs and cats. Surgical treatment for ureterolithiasis has a reported 20–25% perioperative mortality in dogs and cats.

56i. Severe bilateral otitis externa and media resulting in mineralization of the soft tissues in and around the ear canal.

ii. The only surgical option for this patient is a total ear canal ablation and concurrent lateral bulla osteotomy. Lateral bulla osteotomy should always be combined with total ear canal ablation so that all epithelium is removed from the lining of the bulla.

iii. Some dogs will have non-neoplastic disease such as ceruminous hyperplasia, inflammatory polyps and ceruminus gland cysts. The majority of tumors within the external ear canal are malignant and epithelial in origin. The most common malignant tumors found in the external ear canals of dogs are ceruminous gland adenocarcinoma, squamous cell carcinoma, anaplastic carcinoma, soft tissue sarcoma and melanoma. In cats, almost 90% of ear canal tumors are malignant. Ceruminous gland adenocarcinoma, squamous cell carcinoma, sebaceous adeno-carcinoma and anaplastic carcinoma have all been reported.

57 A 13-year-old mixed breed dog presents for increased respiratory effort. A solitary lung mass is diagnosed in the accessory lung lobe (57). An accessory lung lobectomy is planned.
i. What approach is used to perform this surgery?
ii. Describe the surgical procedure.

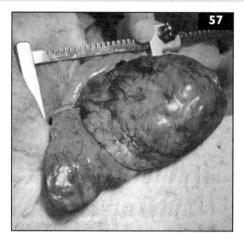

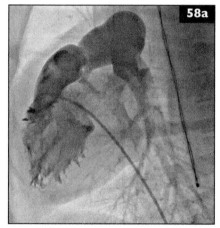

58 A lateral thoracic view of an angiogram of a 6-month-old male Beagle with a grade IV/VI left basilar systolic murmur is shown (58a).
i. Where is the catheter located within the heart?
ii. What is your diagnosis?
iii. What is the most common treatment option for severe cases?
iv. Name two surgical treatment options for severe cases.
v. What is different about Boxers and English Bulldogs with this condition and why is this important?

57i. The accessory lung lobe is a lobe of the right lung. The approach used to remove this lung lobe is a right fifth intercostal approach. The accessory lung lobe is a small lobe that extends from the medial surface of the right lung into the mediastinal recess. It partially passes over the caudal vena cava.

ii. A standard right fifth intercostal thoracotomy is performed. The healthy lung lobes are packed out of the way and the pleura is incised to expose the pulmonary vessels. The lung lobectomy can be performed with ligation or stapling equipment. If ligatures are used, the pulmonary artery is identified and triple ligated with the central ligature placed as a transfixion ligature. The same ligation is performed on the vein. The vessels are transected. The bronchus is cross-clamped, transected and the lung lobe is removed to provide more working room. Horizontal mattress sutures are preplaced across the bronchus and tied. The bronchus is then oversewn with a simple continuous suture pattern. If stapling equipment is used, a thoracoabdominal stapler (30 or 55) is placed across the hilus and fired. The closure of the bronchus is tested for air leaks by instilling the thorax with warm saline and producing 20–30 cm of water pressure within the ventilation system.

58i. The catheter is in the right ventricle (**58b**). The catheter was inserted in the femoral vein, courses through the caudal vena cava, right atrium, across the tricuspid valve and into the right ventricle.

ii. The diagnosis is pulmonic stenosis. There is a filling defect at the level of the abnormal pulmonary valve and a poststenotic dilation of the pulmonary artery.

iii. The most common treatment for severe cases is catheter-based balloon valvuloplasty. This procedure can be performed by gaining access to the jugular vein or femoral vein. A balloon dilation catheter is passed through the venous system, into the right atrium, across the tricuspid valve, into the right ventricle and finally across the pulmonary valve. The balloon dilation catheter is inflated to open the stenotic pulmonary valve and then the catheter is removed.

iv. Surgical options include pulmonic patch-graft valvuloplasty, pulmonic valvotomy or right ventricle to pulmonary artery conduit repair.

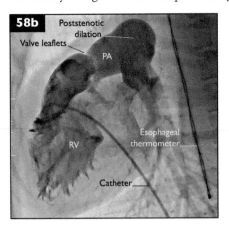

58b Poststenotic dilation. Valve leaflets. PA. Esophageal thermometer. RV. Catheter.

v. Boxers and English Bulldogs (as well as other breeds) can have a concurrent anomalous left main coronary artery. An 'R2A' coronary anomaly is characterized by an anomalous left main coronary artery that arises as a branch from a single right coronary artery. This anomalous left coronary encircles the main pulmonary artery at the level of the stenotic valve and is a contraindication to both standard balloon valvuloplasty and patch-graft valvuloplasty.

59 An 8-year-old spayed, female domestic short hair cat presents for evaluation. Upon physical examination, multifocal areas of exfoliative dermatitis (59a) are noted along with a non-compressible thorax and muffled heart sounds. A lateral thoracic radiograph is provided (59b).

i. What are your differential diagnoses upon review of the thoracic radiograph?

ii. Can additional diagnostic testing help narrow the differential list?

iii. Are the skin lesions related to thoracic abnormality?

iv. What is the prognosis for this cat?

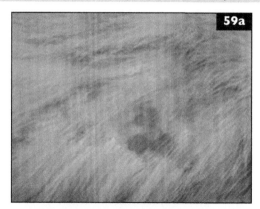

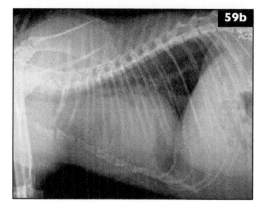

60 An 8-month-old intact, male mixed breed dog presents for weight loss and vomiting. An abdominal ultrasound is performed.

i. What is your diagnosis?

ii. What concurrent conditions are associated with this abnormality?

iii. What additional diagnostics should be performed?

iv. What treatment is recommended?

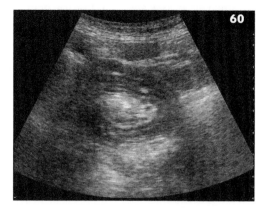

59i. Differential diagnoses include mediastinal lymphoma, thymoma, thymic branchial cyst and granuloma/abscess.

ii. Fine needle aspiration and/or needle core biopsy can be performed – ideally under ultrasound or CT guidance. Cytologic evaluation of thymoma will show abundant small lymphocytes and clusters of epithelial cells. Other inflammatory cells, such as neutrophils and mononuclear cells, may be present. In cases where lymphoma cannot be ruled out, flow cytometry can be used to distinguish between lymphoma and thymoma. A study has shown that 10% or greater small lymphocytes positive for cell surface markers CD4 and CD8 is diagnostic for thymoma.

iii. Yes, exfoliative dermatitis is a paraneoplastic syndrome of thymoma in cats but not in dogs. Other paraneoplastic syndromes in cats include myasthenia gravis (MG) (not as common as in dogs) and polymyositis. Thymoma-associated paraneoplastic syndromes in dogs include MG, polymyositis, myocarditis and humoral hypercalcemia of malignancy.

iv. Prognosis for thymoma in cats is good with a 1- and 3-year survival of 89% and 74%, respectively. A lymphocyte rich subtype of thymoma is positively associated with long-term survival.

60i. This dog has an intussusception. One portion of intestine (the intussusceptum) has invaginated into the lumen of another portion of the intestine (the intussuscipiens).

ii. In young dogs, intussusception is associated with enteritis. Enteritis may occur secondary to viruses (specifically parvovirus), parasites, foreign bodies, cecal inversion or previous surgery. In older animals, intussusception is more commonly reported secondary to intestinal neoplasia. The most common location of intussusception is ileocolic (Rallis, 2000).

iii. Young dogs with intussusception should undergo a test for parvovirus and a fecal flotation examination. Following surgery, appropriate treatment for viral infection or parasitism should be commenced. Older dogs should undergo thoracic radiographs prior to surgery. Intussusception in older animals is associated with intestinal neoplasia and detection of pulmonary metastasis prior to surgery is important for determining prognosis.

iv. Exploratory surgery and surgical reduction or resection of the intussusception is usually required. A thorough abdominal exploratory should be performed as multiple intussusceptions may be detected. Reduction of the intussusception is attempted if the intestine appears viable. If reduction is not possible or if the involved gastrointestinal tract is non-viable, a resection and anastomosis is performed. In older animals, resection and anastomosis, rather than reduction, is recommended because underlying neoplasia is suspected.

61 An 8-year-old, intact, male mixed breed dog with bilateral perineal swelling, tenesmus and constipation presents for investigation for a suspected bilateral perineal hernia.

i. Which procedures would you perform to confirm the diagnosis?

ii. Which ancillary diagnostic tests can be useful?

iii. Standard surgical treatment involves perineal hernia repair using muscle transposition techniques. Which adjunctive surgical procedures to herniorraphy can be used to manage large, recurrent or complicated cases?

iv. Which factors may affect recurrence?

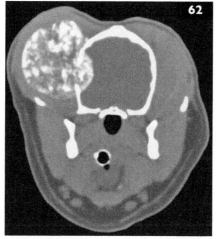

62 A 9-year-old castrated, male Bichon Frise presents for a large, firm swelling on the dorsolateral aspect of the cranium. The mass has been slowly expanding in size for several months. CT of the skull shows a large, spherical mass that is described as having a 'popcorn ball appearance' involving the parietal bone (**62**).

i. What are the differentials for the mass, and which is most likely based on the imaging characteristics?

ii. Name and describe the surgical procedure that is indicated for removal of the mass.

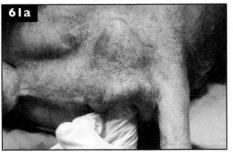

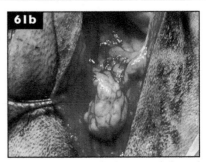

61i. Definitive diagnosis can be made on the basis of clinical findings and digital rectal examination. Rectal examination detects the loss of integrity of the pelvic diaphragm, which is revealed by the visualization of the tip of the index finger through the skin lateral to the anus (**61a**).

ii. Abdominal radiography can be useful to evaluate size of the prostate and position of the urinary bladder. Abdominal ultrasonography may also be useful to evaluate size of the prostate, and contents of the hernia sac. Contrast cystography is occasionally performed to assess integrity of the lower urinary tract and position of the urinary bladder. Barium administration by mouth or as an enema can be utilized to evaluate rectal abnormalities.

iii. Cystopexy and colopexy have been reported as an adjunctive or sole treatment for perineal hernia. These techniques can be performed as staged procedures or concurrent with surgical treatment of the perineal hernia. Several benefits are reported. Cystopexy and colopexy improve visualization of the perineal space by preventing viscera from occupying the hernia (**61b**); this makes repair easier, faster and more accurate. As a consequence, iatrogenic damage to anatomical structures is less likely, and incidence of postoperative fecal incontinence, due to damage to caudal rectal nerve or external anal sphincter, is reduced. Moreover, cystopexy and colopexy improve the prognosis of bilateral and complicated perineal hernias, and allow investigation and treatment of concomitant surgical prostatic disease and retroflexed bladder. The colopexy allows the descending colon and rectum to regain the tubular shape, reduces the rectal diameter and accumulation of feces will diminish. Castration performed at the same time will cause atrophy of the prostate, making the perineal space even wider and patients may return to normal defecation in 2–3 weeks.

iv. Reported recurrence rates range from 0% to 70%. Factors reported to affect recurrence include surgeon experience, previous repairs, suture material, local tissue strength, tension applied to sutures, ongoing predisposing factors and whether the patient is neutered or intact.

62i. Differentials include multilobular osteochondrosarcoma (MLO), osteosarcoma and osteoma. Based on the imaging appearance and description, a MLO tumor of the bone is most likely.

ii. A right sided craniectomy of the parietotemporal bone is indicated for mass removal. With the location extending ventral, the ramus of the mandible may need to be removed to provide access to the mass.

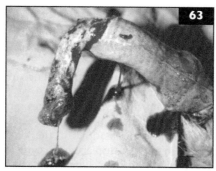

63 A 3-year-old mixed breed dog presents with ventral penile deviation, dysuria, hemorrhage from the penis and urethra and pain and crepitus on palpation of the penis following a dog fight (63).
i. What is the diagnosis?
ii. How common is this condition?
iii. What are the treatment options?

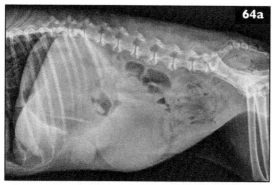

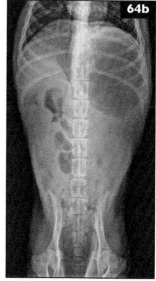

64 An abdominal radiograph of a 6-year-old castrated, male Lhasa Apso is shown (64a, b). The radiograph was made because the owners reported vomiting with increasing frequency over the last several months. The vomitus contains partially digested food and often occurs several hours after feeding. The dog appears otherwise healthy. This radiograph was made after the dog had been fasted 10 hours.
i. What is your diagnosis?
ii. What additional diagnostics could be performed to support your diagnosis?
iii. What surgical procedures could be performed for treatment?

Answers: 63, 64

63i. This dog has a fracture of the os penis and penile laceration. The fracture is palpable but radiographs should be performed to determine os penis damage. Urethral catheterization and retrograde urethrogram should be performed to determine urethral obstruction or perforation.
ii. Fracture of the os penis is an uncommon situation occurring in 2% of the dogs presented with penile and preputial abnormalities.
iii. Management of penile trauma and evaluation of urethral involvement should be initially attempted by passing a urethral catheter to extend beyond the fracture site, followed by radiographic examination of the os penis and retrograde urethrography. In cases of minimally displaced fracture and patent urethra, no treatment is necessary. Otherwise an indwelling catheter is introduced to achieve fracture immobilization for 1–3 weeks. Marked deviation of the os penis may require internal fixation of the fracture with a mini plate. If urethral damage occurs urethral anastomosis may be attempted. If this fails, or in the presence of fractures that accompany massive urethral and penile trauma, partial penile amputation alone or combined with scrotal urethrostomy are required. The owner should be cautioned to monitor urinary habits. Urethral obstruction occurring 2 years following os penis fractures has been reported, due to callus and fibrous tissue proliferation compressing the urethra (Kelly, 1995).

64i. This dog has pyloric outflow obstruction. Pyloric outflow obstructions can be congenital or acquired. Congenital obstructions are usually pyloric muscular hypertrophy. These congenital muscular obstructions typically occur in young (less than 1 year) brachycephalic dogs. Acquired obstructions generally occur in small breed dogs and are either mucosal in origin or a combination of mucosal and muscular. Foreign bodies or neoplasia of the pylorus can also lead to pyloric outflow obstruction.
ii. Abdominal radiographs are suggestive of pyloric outflow obstruction when the stomach is filled with food following an 8-hour or longer fast (in this case, the stomach is filled with fluid and air). Contrast radiography may show an 'apple core' appearance to the pylorus, indicating narrowing at the pylorus when contrast is administered by mouth. The contrast radiography may also be used to prove delayed gastric emptying. Ultrasonography of the stomach, specifically the pylorus, may be helpful. Ultrasonography may show thickening of the gastric layers of the pylorus. Endoscopy may be helpful to diagnose dogs with pyloric stenosis due to mucosal hypertrophy. In these cases, the enlarged mucosal folds are seen in the pyloric outflow tract.
iii. Benign pyloric outflow obstruction can be treated by pyloromyotomy (Fredet–Ramstedt pyloromyotomy), transverse pyloroplasty (Heineke–Mikuliz) or Y–U advancement pyloroplasty. With both pyloroplasty techniques, the lumen of the stomach is entered, facilitating full thickness pyloric biopsies. Full thickness biopsies should always be acquired in order to diagnose neoplasia if present. If neoplasia is present and confined to the pylorus, a Billroth I (pylorectomy with gastroduodenal anastomosis) is indicated.

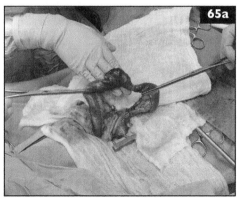
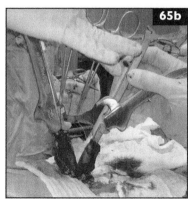

65 A 12-year-old castrated, male mixed breed dog presents for an intestinal mass. Abdominal exploration is unremarkable aside from the isolated mass.

i. What instruments are being used to occlude the intestinal lumen and isolate the intestinal mass (**65a**)?

ii. What instrument is being used to perform the anastomosis after the mass was removed (**65b**)? What type of anastomosis does this instrument perform? What two staple size options does this stapler have and what shape are these staples when closed and why?

iii. If suture were used instead of staples, what is the preferred suture pattern? What type of suture is recommended and how far apart should each suture be?

66 An 11-year-old German Shepherd dog presents for exploratory laparotomy and liver biopsies. The dog has low body condition, low albumin and glucose, severe elevation of ALP, ALT and cholesterol. The dog has been vomiting throughout the night. You want to have a quick recovery from anesthesia and also to provide adequate, balanced anesthesia utilizing a pure μ-opioid. You must decide between the following opioids: butorphanol, hydromorphone, fentanyl or remifentanil.

i. Which will be the best option?

ii. Why is this the best option?

iii. What other consideration should you have in mind when using this particular drug?

65i. The instruments are Doyen intestinal forceps. Doyen forceps are atraumatic to prevent damaging the intestinal loops. The grooves on Doyen forceps are longitudinal and the tips can either be straight or curved. In this photograph, one is applied orally and one aborally. The intestine is transected leaving the Doyen in place to prevent spillage of gastrointestinal contents.

ii. The instrument is a reusable gastrointestinal anastomosis (GIA) stapler. The GIA stapler performs an antiperistaltic side-to-side anastomosis (functional end-to-end). Available GIA staple cartridge lengths are 50 mm and 90 mm. Reusable GIA instruments are only available with 3.8 mm staples that close to a height of 1.5 mm. The staples have a 3.0 mm crown width (Tobias, 2007). The staples close in a 'B' shape, which allows for blood flow through the staple openings.

iii. The preferred suture pattern for intestinal anastomoses is a single layer of appositional sutures. Appositional patterns include simple interrupted, simple continuous and modified Gambee. One of these patterns should be performed using fine (3-0 or 4-0) absorbable suture material such as polydioxanone or polyglecaprone 25. Each throw should be approximately 3–5 mm from the edge of the tissue and 3–5 mm apart, with additional sutures as needed following a leak check with saline.

66i. Butorphanol is a κ-agonist μ-antagonist, hydromorphone is a μ-opioid but it tends to stimulate vomiting initially. Fentanyl is a short-acting μ-opioid but when administered as an infusion it tends to accumulate in the tissues, prolonging its time of action. The best option in this case would be remifentanil, an ultra-short-acting, pure μ-opioid analog of fentanyl that produces similar effect.

ii. Remifentanil is a potent analgesic and similar to fentanyl. It is able to reduce the requirement of inhalants by 70–75% when used at the high end of the recommended doses as continuous rate infusion (0.8 µg/kg/min). Remifentanil has a short contex-sensitive half-time that, along with a terminal half-life of 4–8 min, the lack of accumulation in tissues and the weak potency of its metabolites, allows its effect to disappear rapidly after discontinuing the infusion thus allowing a faster recovery. Remifentanil is metabolized by non-specific plasma and tissue esterases. Therefore, its elimination is independent of liver function. Using balanced anesthesia allows preservation of liver perfusion better than in situations where high doses of inhalants are used. Time of ambulation after receiving infusion of remifentanil has been reported to be shorter than 22 minutes in dogs suffering liver disease, anesthetized in order to obtain liver biopsies (Anagnostou, 2011).

iii. Bradycardia is the most common side-effect reported which occurs through a central vagal effect. In addition, respiratory depression has been reported during remifentanil use. Since its effects disappear quickly after stopping the infusion, analgesia should be administered close to its discontinuation.

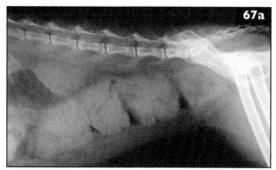

67 A 10-year-old domestic medium hair cat presents for a 3-month history of tenesmus and constipation. Radiographs of the abdomen were obtained (67a).
i. What is the radiographic diagnosis?
ii. What is the purported etiopathogenesis for this condition?
iii. Describe potential treatment options for this cat.
iv. What is the prognosis following surgical intervention?

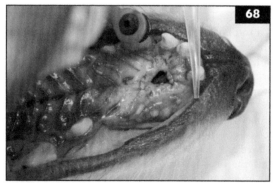

68 A photograph of an oronasal fistula is shown (68). This dog experienced trauma to the face approximately 3 months prior to the photograph.
i. What are the two main categories of oronasal fistulas?
ii. What are some closure options for oronasal fistulas?

67i. Megacolon

ii. Idiopathic megacolon is the most common form of acquired megacolon in cats. The exact cause of idiopathic megacolon is unclear; however, behavioral (refusal to defecate) reasons or abnormalities in either the intrinsic or extrinsic nerve supply to colonic smooth muscle are implicated. Secondary megacolon may occur due to prolonged mechanical obstruction of the distal colon and rectum due to a functional

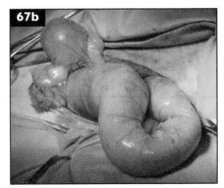

abnormality of the anorectal area, healed pelvic fracture, foreign body, intramural or extramural mass or neurologic disease such as dysautonomia or lumbosacral spinal cord disease.

iii. Cats with chronic constipation may be treated conservatively with intravenous fluids, multiple enemas, dietary modification and osmotic laxatives. Prokinetics, such as cisapride, may be useful if irreversible changes are not present. Underlying mechanical obstruction should be addressed if present. If conservative therapy fails, surgical intervention may be warranted. If the ileum and ileocecocolic valve are normal, a subtotal colectomy (colocolostomy) may be performed (**67b**). If the ileocecocolic junction is abnormal, or if significant tension is present on the anastomosis site, a total colectomy (ileocolic anastomosis) may be warranted.

iv. Feces usually remain soft after colocolic anastomosis. Diarrhea is often present after removal of the ileocecocolic junction, but usually resolves to soft feces. Up to 45% of cats with the idiopathic form of the disease demonstrate recurrence of clinical signs that may require treatment.

68i. Oronasal fistulas are categorized into healed and non-healed. Healed oronasal fistulas have mucosal continuity between the oral and nasal cavities. Non-healed oronasal fistulas have not yet formed a continuous mucosa.

ii. Closure options for oronasal fistulas are divided into two broad categories: single flap closure and double flap closure. A single flap of gingival mucosa and buccal mucosa is a good option for smaller fistulas. Alternatively, mucoperiosteum from the hard palate can be elevated and transposed to cover the defect. The mucoperiosteum would not be a good option in this case as the defect is on midline and a portion of the tissue desired for the closure has been damaged in the disease process.

   Double flap closures can be utilized both for healed and non-healed fistulas. In double flap techniques, mucosa is provided to close the oral and nasal surfaces.

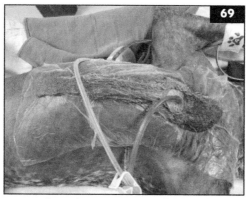

69 A 5-year-old neutered, male German Shorthaired Pointer presents with a stick-puncture wound to the thorax. After initial wound treatment, including exploratory thoracotomy, copious lavage and sharp debridement of foreign debris, you elect to perform delayed wound closure and place a vacuum assisted closure (VAC) bandage (**69**).
i. What are four advantages of using this type of wound management?
ii. What is the optimal pressure that should be used in VAC treatment?
iii. How frequently must a VAC bandage be changed?
iv. What are four contraindications for use of VAC treatment?

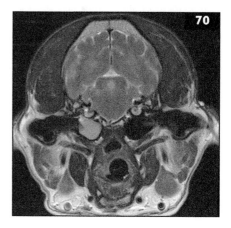

70 A 3-year-old spayed, female Cocker Spaniel is admitted for an acute onset of vomiting, circling to the right and a right head tilt. Based on your neurologic exam, you diagnose right peripheral vestibular disease. An MRI is performed, and the patient is diagnosed with otitis media/interna (**70**). The dog has a history of recurrent ear infections.
i. What are other differentials for the clinical signs in this dog?
ii. What are the criteria for surgical intervention in this dog?
iii. What surgical procedures could be performed?

69i. VAC, also known as negative pressure wound therapy, applies a uniform subatmospheric pressure to a wound, providing several well documented benefits including: decreased formation of interstitial edema or seroma, stimulation of neovascularization, enhanced formation of granulation tissue, improved bacterial clearance and hastened second intention wound closure. Because of the consistent active drainage, VAC bandages do not have to be changed as frequently as traditional dressings used during the inflammatory phase of healing.

ii. Studies in animals have found that −125 mmHg is the optimal pressure to stimulate angiogenesis and cellular proliferation. This is the recommended setting when VAC is used over open wounds.

iii. VAC bandages should be changed every 48–72 hours. If left *in situ* longer than 72 hours, granulation tissue growth into the foam is a likely complication.

iv. VAC does not provide substantial wound debridement and thus traditional debridement techniques and basic wound care must take place prior to and in addition to VAC therapy. VAC therapy should not be used over necrotic or devitalized tissue. VAC foam should not be placed directly over large blood vessels or nerves. VAC therapy should not be used in a neoplastic wound bed as neovascularization and cellular proliferation are documented effects of VAC therapy. VAC should not be used in patients with coagulopathies or active bleeding from the wound.

70i. Other differentials include primary secretory otitis media, nasopharyngeal polyp or aural cholesteatoma. Idiopathic vestibular disease would be possible had the MRI examination been normal.

ii. Cases that require surgery are those that are considered refractory to medical management or those that have multiple relapses of infection. This includes cases that do not respond to appropriate antibiotic therapy as well as cases that have proliferative tissue or stenotic ear canals that makes administration of topical medications difficult.

iii. Procedures include total ear canal ablation with bulla osteotomy (TECABO), ear canal resection and ventral bulla osteotomy. In this case, a TECABO would be appropriate because of the breed; Cocker Spaniels have notoriously difficult to manage otitis and thus Cocker Spaniels with recurrent otitis externa are treated with TECABO.

71 An 8-year-old spayed, female Toy Poodle is presented for a 'goose-honk' cough of increasing severity and frequency over a 1-year period. Tracheal collapse is identified on plain radiographs of the cervical and thoracic region. Extraluminal prosthetic tracheal rings are placed.
i. Name the common indications for this surgical procedure.
ii. Describe the surgical procedure, including methods for skeletonizing the trachea.
iii. Name several complications associated with this surgical procedure.

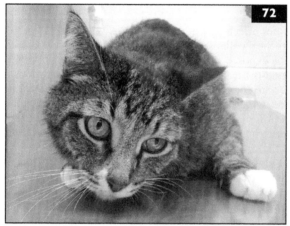

72 A 9-year-old castrated, male domestic short hair cat presents for progressive head tilt and lethargy (72). The owners report the cat has been shaking his head on occasion as well as scratching at the left ear. On physical examination, the head is tilted. CT imaging identifies soft tissue opacity completely filling the left tympanic bulla with extension into the external ear canal, as well as fluid accumulation in the region of the inner ear. Biopsy confirms an inflammatory polyp.
i. This is a somewhat odd presentation of inflammatory polyp in this cat – why? What is the typical signalment for feline inflammatory polyps?
ii. Inflammatory polyps can originate from two locations; what are they? What differences in presentation would be noted based on polyp origin?
iii. Surgical removal is the therapeutic option of choice for inflammatory polyps. What other options for treatment are available?

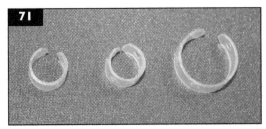

71i. Surgical intervention is considered in animals that have failed appropriate medical management, as successful control of clinical signs is expected in 71%. Extraluminal prosthetic rings are used in dogs with collapse restricted to the cervical trachea and thoracic inlet. Median survival time (>4 years) after ring placement was not affected in a cohort of dogs where 33% had a component of intrathoracic tracheal collapse (Becker, 2012) (**71**).

ii. The trachea is exposed through a ventral midline skin incision. Tracheal rings are passed around the trachea, starting caudal to the cricoid. Passage of the rings axially to the recurrent laryngeal nerves is facilitated by skeletonizing the right pedicle, as there is increased space between the trachea and the right recurrent laryngeal nerve. Alternatively, a tunnel is made only where the ring is to be passed. The rings are secured with simple interrupted sutures that encircle the cartilaginous rings and enter the tracheal lumen.

iii. Laryngeal paralysis occurs in 11–30% due to iatrogenic damage during dissection or chronic contact with a prosthetic ring. Tracheal necrosis secondary to skeletonization of the segmental blood supply. Pneumothorax or pneumomediastinum results from inadvertent penetration of the pleura.

72i. Polyps typically present in very young animals, often in cats less than 3 years of age. The advanced age in this cat is atypical, although inflammatory polyps are occasionally diagnosed in older animals. The unilateral involvement is typical.

ii. Polyps can originate from the Eustachian tubes or from the lining of the tympanic bulla. If they originate from the Eustachian tubes, growth tends to progress towards the oropharynx below the soft palate; typical presentation may include upper respiratory signs such as dyspnea, wheezing and stertor. Dysphagia and voice changes may also be noted. If the polyp originates from the middle ear, signs mimic otitis externa/media including head shaking, head tilt, nystagmus and vestibular disease. Exudate within the external canal is also typically reported.

iii. Traction and avulsion can be effective for polyp removal; however, care must be taken to grasp the polyp as close to the base of the pedunculated stalk as possible. Residual tissue can lead to polyp regrowth. Endoscopic removal has been shown to be effective in some cases; this method is similar to traction and avulsion with enhanced visualization and improved location of the polyp base. Laser ablation may also be beneficial, but may be more difficult and time consuming for larger masses.

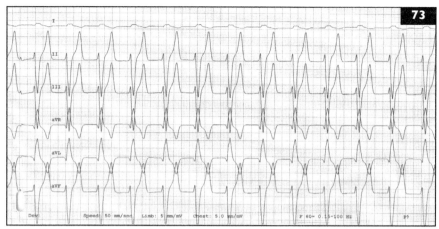

73 An ECG tracing from a 5-year-old castrated, male Great Dane that is recovering from gastric dilatation and volvulus (GDV) surgery is shown (73).
i. What is your ECG rhythm diagnosis?
ii. What are some potential causes of this rhythm abnormality in this case?
iii. What, if any, treatment should be initiated?

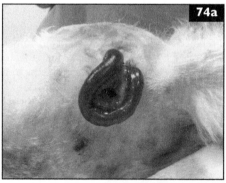

74 A 4-year-old Pomeranian presents after being attacked by another dog (74a).
i. What is the most common cause of evisceration?
ii. What emergency procedures should be performed prior to surgery?
iii. What will surgery involve?

Answers: 73, 74

73i. Accelerated idioventricular rhythm. This is a ventricular rhythm based on the wide and bizarre QRS morphology with lack of associated p waves. The heart rate at ~150 bpm is too slow to be considered ventricular tachycardia.

ii. Ventricular arrhythmias, such as ventricular premature contractions (VPCs), accelerated idioventricular rhythm or ventricular tachycardia, are common in dogs with GDV, even following surgical correction. Electrolyte disturbances, pain, inadequate perfusion, and circulating cardiac depressant factors are potential causes in a case such as this one. Often there is no underlying cardiac disease present. Other causes of this abnormal rhythm can include splenic disease, pancreatitis, immune-mediated diseases, prostatitis, neurologic disease and trauma.

iii. Treatment involves correction of the underlying cause if one can be identified – surgical correction of GDV, correction of electrolyte or acid/base abnormalities if present and improving perfusion. If the ventricular rate increases and is considered ventricular tachycardia, particularly if there is evidence of R-on-T phenomenon, or if there is evidence of hemodynamic compromise such as hypotension or pulse deficits, then anti-arrhythmic therapy with lidocaine is warranted. Typically, accelerated idioventricular rhythms will spontaneously resolve within 2–3 days following GDV surgery.

74i. In veterinary medicine, the most common cause of evisceration injuries is postoperative dehiscence of an abdominal incision.

ii. Preoperative treatment includes hemodynamic stabilization, antimicrobial treatment, extension of the abdominal rent (if needed to prevent strangulation of the eviscerated organs) and application of a sterile covering until surgery is performed.

iii. During surgery, organ viability must be assessed. The eviscerated organs must be cleaned, repaired and replaced in the peritoneal cavity. A full exploratory should be

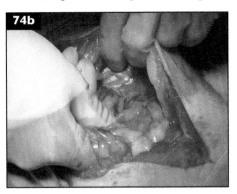

performed to detect other damage. In this case, the abdominal exploratory and reduction of the hernia were performed through a ventral midline incision (**74b**). A copious abdominal lavage should be performed. The abdominal rent should be assessed. Wound edges should be debrided if necessary and the rent should be closed. In this case, the abdominal rent was draped into the surgical field and the rent was closed in the same procedure.

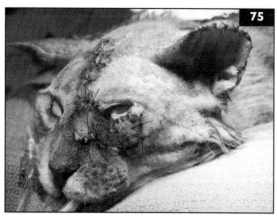

75 A 12-year-old cat presents for a crusting, non-healing lesion on the lower eyelid. A biopsy was performed and is consistent with squamous cell carcinoma. Surgery is performed to remove the lesion and the photograph taken postoperatively (75).
i. What is the name of the skin flap used here?
ii. How is the cornea protected after resection of the lower eyelid?
iii. This technique is appropriate if what percentage of the lower eyelid is involved?
iv. What technique should be utilized for smaller lesions?

76 An 11-year-old neutered, male Beagle mix presents for evaluation of pollakiuria, stranguria and intermittent urinary incontinence. Frank blood is observed at the end of urination. The patient is otherwise in good health.
i. Which portion of the urogenital tract is the most likely source of hematuria?
ii. Which tumor types most commonly affect the urinary tract?
iii. Ultrasound findings raise your index of suspicion for neoplasia. Which methods can be utilized to collect samples for cytology and/or histopathology?

75i. The pictured skin flap is a transposition flap. In a transposition flap, the defect and the flap share a border. In this case, they share the medial margin. Transposition flaps rotate on a pivot point. Commonly, the transposition flap is rotated within 90 degrees of the wound's axis but can be pivoted up to 180 degrees.
ii. During this procedure, a third eyelid lateral advancement is performed (Schmide, 2005). The lateralized third eyelid provides a continuous conjunctival surface against the cornea. The third eyelid is lateralized and the superficial conjunctival surface is scarified. After scarification, the raised transposition flap is sutured to the third eyelid and remaining skin edge (Schmide, 2005).
iii. If the full thickness defect in the lower lid is between 33% and 100% of the eyelid margin, this procedure is appropriate.
iv. Full thickness lower eyelid defects can be directly apposed and sutured if the defect is less than one-third of the eyelid margin. The lateral canthal ligament can be divided to relieve eyelid tension during direct closure if necessary. Wider defects may require an advancement flap.

76i. When bleeding is associated with lesions in the urinary bladder and prostate, blood is most commonly observed at the end of urination. Blood noted at the beginning of urination is typically associated with disease affecting the penis, prepuce, vagina, vulva, urethra or prostate, and will typically dissipate during urination. Bleeding noted uniformly throughout micturition is more likely associated with disease affecting the kidneys, ureters or urinary bladder.
ii. Transitional cell carcinoma (TCC) is the most common primary tumor to form in the urinary bladder. Other differentials include leiomyoma, leiomyosarcoma, squamous cell carcinoma and rhabdomyosarcoma.
iii. While TCC typically involves the trigone of the urinary bladder in the dog and often the apex of the urinary bladder in cat, any portion of the urinary tract can be affected. Free catch urine samples can be used for cytology. Traumatic catheterization (blind, palpation-guided or ultrasound-guided) can be used to collect samples for cytology and often histopathology. Cystoscopy provides visualization of the urethra and urinary bladder and can facilitate collection of samples. Surgical biopsies can also be collected. Ultrasound-guided fine needle aspiration or biopsy is contraindicated due to the exfoliative nature of TCC and risk for potential seeding of tumor in the abdomen.

77 A 5-year-old castrated, male German Shepherd dog presents for a history of progressive perianal irritation and straining to defecate. The owner has reported that the dog will frequently lick at his hind end, under the tail, and scoot along the carpet. Although diarrhea has not been noted, the owner describes the dog's stool as rather soft and with a ribbon-like appearance. On physical examination, the following lesions are noted (77).

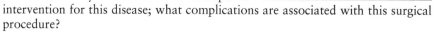

i. What is the name for this condition?
ii. In which breeds of dogs is it most commonly reported?
iii. En bloc surgical removal used to be the most commonly recommended therapeutic intervention for this disease; what complications are associated with this surgical procedure?
iv. What alternative options for therapeutic intervention are available?

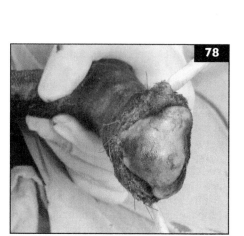

78 A 12-year–old mixed breed dog presents with sloughing of all digits of the left hind limb associated with a thromboembolic abnormality. In view of the poor ability for ambulation related to a possible limb amputation, the dog underwent a salvage procedure to save the paw (78).
i. Name this surgical procedure.
ii. What are the indications for performing this type of paw reconstruction?
iii. Describe the procedure.

77i. Perianal fistula (PAF) (anal furunculosis).

ii. German Shepherd dogs are most commonly affected; however, other breeds with low carried, broad based tails (e.g. Irish Setter, Labrador Retriever, Collies) may also be at risk for lesion development.

iii. Complications included anal stricture or stenosis, fecal incontinence, poor wound healing and recurrence of fistula lesions.

iv. Medical management of PAF lesions is often effective, leading to complete resolution of clinical signs. Recurrence of fistula lesions is still possible with therapy; many patients require continued life-long medical management. Perianal hygiene is recommended for all patients including clipping of excess hair and bathing with topical antiseptic solution (e.g. dilute chlorhexidine). If secondary bacterial infection is present, systemic antibiotherapy may be indicated. Although the influence of food allergy with regard to lesion development is questionable, some patients may respond to elimination diet trials (e.g. hydrolyzed or novel protein diets) or other dietary manipulation. Cyclosporine (with or without concurrent ketoconazole) has been highly beneficial for management of lesions; response is often seen within 4 months of administration. Topical tacrolimus is also effective when applied once or twice daily. This may be initiated once more severe lesions are relatively healed. Prednisone administration is beneficial for most patients; however, higher doses (1–2 mg/kg daily, then tapered) are typically required and side-effects of long-term administration are concerning. Other alternative therapies include cryotherapy, laser excision or chemical cauterization. As with en bloc resection, multiple procedures may be required.

78i. Pandigital amputation and metatarsal pad advancement.

ii. Metatarsal pad advancement is performed when loss of all digits of a limb occurs. The digits may lose their viability as a result of thromboembolism associated with trap injury, pressure necrosis and other traumatic causes, immune-mediated vasculopathy and phlebitis.

iii. To perform such type of surgery the metatarsal or metacarpal pad should remain intact. A transverse incision is made in the dorsal paw surface proximal to the demarcation line, if present. The incision is continued in the plantar paw surface cranial to the metatarsal or metacarpal pad. All the digits are disarticulated at the level of metatarsophalangeal or metacarpophalangeal junction and the distal metatarsal and metacarpal bones are resected for proper pad accommodation. The pad is advanced and sutured to the paw stump under the bones with tension relieving sutures. A Penrose drain was placed in this case.

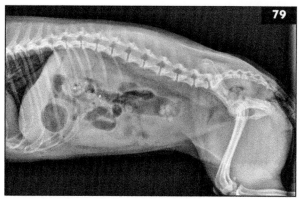

79 A cystotomy was performed in a 3-year-old spayed, female mixed breed dog. An abdominal radiograph is available for review (**79**). At surgery, uroliths were removed from the bladder and submitted for stone analysis. Concurrently, a urine culture was performed and was positive for bacterial growth.

i. What is the most likely stone type?
ii. What is the most likely type of bacteria causing the infection and leading to the development of this stone type?

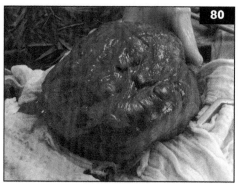

80 A 10-year-old spayed, female German Shepherd dog presents for a decreased appetite, weight loss, lethargy and a distended abdomen. At surgery, a mass is found arising from the colon (**80**).

i. What are differential diagnoses for this mass?
ii. What is the 'lag phase' of healing in reference to the intestinal tract? When does this lag phase occur and when is the most likely time for surgical dehiscence?
iii. Aside from dehiscence, what are the four most common complications associated with large intestinal tumor removal?

79i. Struvite (magnesium ammonium phosphate) stones are the most likely stone type in this dog. Overall, struvite and calcium oxalate are the two most common stones removed from the bladder of dogs. About 53% of stones submitted from dogs contain struvite while about 42% contain calcium oxalate (Low, 2010). Given that this dog has a urinary tract infection, struvite becomes more likely. Struvite stones are radiopaque and are often found in the face of urinary tract infection.

ii. Infection with urease-producing organisms is required for infection-induced uroliths to form. Urease-producing organisms include *Staphylococcus* species, *Proteus* species, *Streptococcus* species, *Klebsiella* species and *Ureaplasma* species. These urease-producing bacteria are able to hydrolize urea into ammonia, bicarbonate and carbonate. The result is an increase in urine pH and urinary supersaturation (Westropp, 2010). The ammonia is changed to ammonium, which becomes available for the formation of magnesium ammonioum phosphate (struvite).

In cats, struvite stone formation usually occurs in sterile urine. The urine becomes supersaturated and uroliths form. Alternatively, struvite stones may be present in sterile urine or in urine infected with non-urease-producing bacteria. In these cases, urinary tract infection is not the cause of struvite formation.

80i. Up to 60% of intestinal tumors arise from the large intestine. A majority of these large intestinal tumors are malignant. Differentials for the large intestinal mass include adenocarcinoma, lymphosarcoma, gastrointestinal stromal tumor and gastrointestinal leiomyosarcoma.

ii. The 'lag phase' of healing includes the first 1–4 days after surgery. Immediately after surgical closure, a fibrin clot forms. This clot will be the initial barrier, along with the suture line, to prevent leakage of intestinal contents. White blood cells infiltrate the area and neutrophils are the predominant cell type at the surgical wound for the first 2–3 days. Neutrophils are then replaced by macrophages as the most abundant white blood cell. During this early time of healing, collagen synthesis and collagen degradation are occurring concurrently. This concurrent degradation and synthesis of collagen during the first 3–5 days after surgery makes this time period the most likely for surgical dehiscence to occur. This means that the sutures or staples placed in the colon provide the main holding strength at the surgery site in the early postoperative period.

iii. The most common complications include hemorrhage, diarrhea, fecal incontinence, infection and stricture. Stricture is more likely to occur when using a single or double layer inverting pattern. For this reason, appositional suture patterns are preferred.

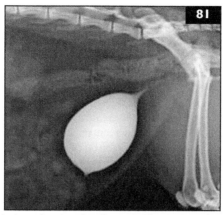

81 i. What diagnostic imaging test has been performed in this cat (**81**)?
ii. What is your diagnosis based on this test?
iii. What clinical variations of this/these conditions are described?
iv. What is the recommended treatment for symptomatic pets?

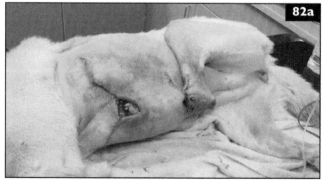

82 An 8-year-old Korean Jindo presents with a degloving injury to the left distal pelvic limb in the region of the metatarsals. The wound is grossly infected. After managing the wound for 1 week until a healthy granulation tissue bed is present, you decided to perform the procedure pictured (**82a**).
i. What is the pictured procedure?
ii. How should the flap be developed to avoid ischemic damage?
iii. What are two other options for closure of a distal pelvic limb defect?

81i. A positive contrast cystogram has been performed in this cat. This study can be used to identify congenital bladder abnormalities, bladder rupture, radiolucent bladder calculi and bladder masses.

ii. This cat has a vesicourachal diverticulum. This occurs when the external opening of the urachus closes but a diverticulum remains at the apex of the bladder.

iii. Vesicourachal diverticuli may occur as macroscopic or microscopic forms. These congenital abnormalities are often incidental findings.

iv. Complications associated with vesicourachal diverticulum often include recurrent urinary tract infections. Animals with recurrent urinary tract infections can be considered 'symptomatic' and surgery can be recommended. The recommended surgery is partial cystectomy with excision of the vesicourachal diverticulum.

82i. The procedure pictured is a distant direct flap utilizing the tissue of the lateral abdomen.

ii. This flap should be elevated and the recipient site introduced. The flap can be formed either as a hinge (single pedicle) or pouch (bipedicle – pictured here). After introduction of the recipient site, the skin edges are sutured to the wound margins. The animal is bandaged to prevent motion between the wound and the flap. After 10–14 days, the pedicle(s) are divided. The pedicle(s) should be divided in stages by releasing one-half to one-third every 2 or 3 days to avoid ischemic injury (**82b**). For successful survival of the flap, revascularization between the recipient bed and overlying dermal surface of the flap must occur.

iii. Distal pelvic limb defects may also be addressed by use of indirect/delayed tubed flap, a reverse saphenous conduit flap or a free graft. Due to the time, expense and the need for multiple surgical procedures increasing the likelihood of complications and flap necrosis, axial pattern flaps and free grafts have replaced the need for most tube flaps.

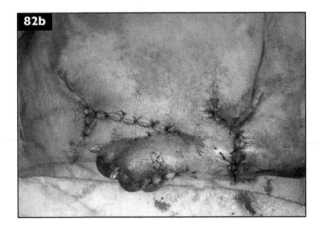

82b

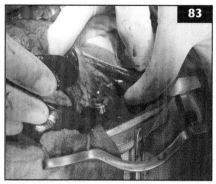

83 A 6-month-old female Miniature Schnauzer presents for blindness. The dog is reportedly very small compared to her littermates and has always been quiet. Recently, she has begun to display abnormal activity that occurs shortly after feeding.

i. What is your diagnosis (83)?
ii. What changes on screening blood work might be associated with this disease?
iii. List five different surgical techniques that could be utilized for treatment.
iv. What medications would you prescribe this dog for treatment prior to surgery?

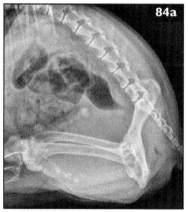

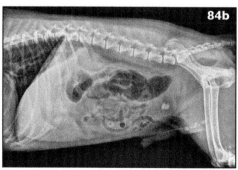

84 A lateral abdominal radiograph of an 8-year-old male dog presenting for lethargy, vomiting, decreased appetite and inability to urinate is shown (84a, b).
i. What is your diagnosis?
ii. What other tests would you like to perform?
iii. What treatment would you recommend?

83i. Congenital extrahepatic portosystemic shunt.

ii. On CBC you may observe microcytosis, with approximately 70% of dogs having a documented normochromic, non-regenerative anemia. Typically microcytosis resolves after shunt attenuation. Target cells may be seen in dogs. Leukocytosis may occur due to inadequate hepatic endotoxin and bacteria clearance from portal circulation and subsequent increased antigenic stimulation.

On chemistry panel, deficiencies associated with decreased hepatic synthesis are commonly seen and include hypoalbuminemia (50%), decreased BUN (70%), hypocholesterolemia and hypoglycemia. Mild increases in serum liver enzyme activities (ALT and ALP) are also common. Urinalysis abnormalities include decreased urine specific gravity and the presence of ammonium biurate crystalluria. Bile acids or ammonia level testing are recommended to evaluate liver function.

iii. Reported methods for surgical occlusion of portosystemic shunts include: (1) placement of an ameroid constrictor; (2) cellophane banding; (3) hydraulic occluder; (4) ligation with silk suture; and (5) intravascular occlusion with thrombogenic coils.

iv. Most patients should undergo medical management for a minimum of 14 days prior to undergoing anesthesia for diagnostic procedures or surgical occlusion. Underweight patients may benefit from longer pretreatment. Lactulose promotes acidification of colonic contents, entrapping luminal ammonia as ammonium. Lactulose also speeds colonic evacuation. Antibiotics, such as neomycin, can be administered to decrease colonic bacterial numbers. Nutritional management is particularly important in young animals or those with extremely poor body condition. Proteins should be moderately restricted. Anticonvulsants may be given to dogs with neurologic abnormalities.

84i. This dog has calculi located in the urinary bladder and urethra. Several calculi are within the penile urethra at the base of the os penis. The base of the os penis is a typical location for stones to become lodged in male dogs, leading to urinary obstruction.

ii. Bloodwork, including CBC and serum biochemistry profile, should be performed. A urinalysis and urine culture should be performed. Bladder mucosa and crushed stone should be collected at surgery for culture. Following removal, the stones should be sent for stone analysis.

iii. The urethral stones should be flushed into the bladder using urohydropulsion. The stones can then be removed through a cystotomy incision. If retropulsion is impossible, either urethrotomy incision or scrotal urethrostomy can be performed. The nephroliths should only be removed if they are causing obstruction or if infection is present. The timing of these procedures should be determined by the health of the dog. A dog with prerenal azotemia should be rehydrated. Dogs with postrenal azotemia may be managed with placement of an indwelling urinary catheter until the azotemia is corrected and then surgery may be performed.

85 An 11-year-old spayed, female Boxer presents for restlessness and panting. A mass is detected on abdominal palpation. The dog's initial PCV is 48%, and TP 7.4 g/dL. An abdominal ultrasound is performed (85a) which identifies an intra-abdominal, cavitated mass of undetermined origin. Fluid is obtained from the center of the mass and cytologic

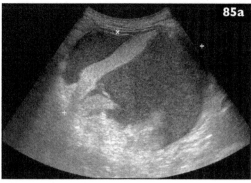

examination yields a PCV of 12%, TP 5 g/dL with a predominance of segmented neutrophils without toxic changes. No intra- or extracellular bacteria are detected. A CBC/chemistry has the following abnormalities: WBC 34,300, with 31,899 segmented neutrophils, 686 lymphocytes and 1715 monocytes.

i. What further diagnostics could be performed to further diagnose this lesion?
ii. What are your differentials for the lesion shown?
iii. What is your surgical recommendation/approach for the lesion?

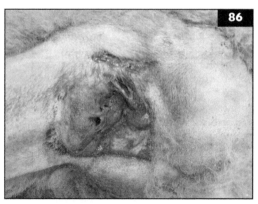

86 A 6-year-old male German Shepherd dog presents with a 1-year history of discomfort and licking of the perianal region (86).
i. What is your diagnosis?
ii. What concurrent medical conditions have been associated with this disease, and what would be your initial therapy for this condition?
iii. If medical therapy is unsuccessful what surgical therapies have been described to deal with the above condition?
iv. What is the long-term prognosis?

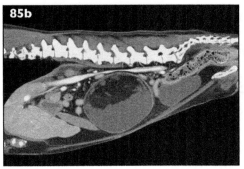

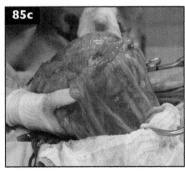

85i. A CT scan could be performed to further delineate the origin of the mass, potential vascular or local invasion and/or the presence of foreign bodies associated with the mass (**85b**). A fine needle aspirate could be performed in order to determine the cell of origin. A true cut biopsy could be performed in order to determine a histologic diagnosis of the mass.

ii. Differential diagnoses that should be considered are: foreign material (Gossypiboma or retained sponge), necrotic lymph node, necrotic solid liver mass, necrotic lipoma and chronic splenic torsion.

iii. The mass does not appear to be locally invasive, does not appear to be involving any of the major intra-abdominal organs based on CT and most likely is originating from the omentum. An intraoperative image (**85c**) shows the mass (a necrotic lipoma) originating from the omentum.

86i. Perianal fistulas (PAFs); also, known as anal furunculosis, perianal sinuses, perianal fistulae, perirectal fistulae and fistula in-ano.

ii. PAFs have been associated with inflammatory bowel disease, eosinophilic colitis and immune mediated proctitis. Medical management of the condition is aimed at immunosuppression of the patient. Immunosuppressive prednisone has been effective for resolving lesions but creates significant side-effects. Oral cyclosporine A either alone or in combination with ketoconazole is an effective therapy for PAF, but has side-effects associated with hepatic and renal toxicity. Topical tacrolimus is efficacious and less expensive, but topical therapy is sometimes resented by the animal and considered distasteful by the owner.

iii. Since PAF may cause damage to the anal sacs, recurrence of fistulas often mandates removal of remnants of the remaining anal sacs. Fistulectomy of the non-healing tracts can be performed either with sharp dissection or using Nd:YAG or CO_2 lasers. Deroofing (saucerization) and fulguration using electrocoagulation or cryotherapy often lead to secondary anal stenosis. Revision anoplasty for anal stenosis commonly will lead to fecal incontinence. High tail amputation, known as caudectomy, has been shown to improve the severity of the fistulas but does not provide resolution.

iv. Currently, medical management is the treatment of choice and many dogs live comfortably for years.

87 An 8-month-old intact, female Doberman Pinscher presents on emergency for a small bowel obstruction.
i. How is von Willebrand disease (VWD) diagnosed?
ii. What are the three different subtypes of VWD?
iii. How is VWD treated?

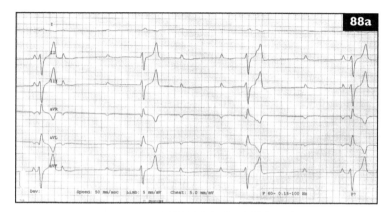

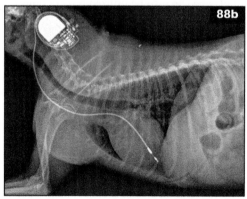

88 An ECG tracing (**88a**) from a 7-year-old castrated, male Cocker Spaniel with an acute history of collapse episodes is shown. A lateral thoracic radiograph from the same dog following treatment is shown (**88b**).
i. Based on the ECG tracing, what is your diagnosis?
ii. What treatment was performed in the Cocker Spaniel?
iii. When is this treatment indicated in dogs?
iv. What was the approach used in the Cocker Spaniel?
v. Where is the tip located within the heart?

87i. A definitive diagnosis of VWD requires measurement of von Willebrand factor (VWF). To classify subtype, quantitative, functional and qualitative VWF assays are required. Screening tests that can be performed in hospital include platelet count, coagulation times and buccal mucosal bleeding times (BMBTs). Platelet function assays (PFAs) can also be performed. Affected individuals will have normal platelet counts and coagulation times but long BMBT and platelet function assay (PFA) closure times.

ii.

Type	Disease severity	VWF concentration	Multimer distribution
Type 1	Mild to moderate	Low	Normal
Type 2	Moderate to severe	Variable reduction	Disproportionate loss of high molecular weight multimers
Type 3	Severe	Total lack of VWF	N/A

iii. Desmopressin acetate (DDAVP) can be used preoperatively (within 30 minutes) in animals with type 1 VWD, as it has been shown to shorten BMBT and PFA-100 closure times. DDAVP stimulates the release of VWF from endothelial cells. Cryoprecipitate is the most effective way of providing high concentrations of VWF rapidly. Fresh frozen plasma can also be utilized but contains a smaller amount of active VWF.

88i. This ECG demonstrates third-degree (complete) atrioventricular (AV) block with a ventricular escape rhythm. It is complete AV block because there are no p waves that are conducted, thus the atrial rate and ventricular rate are completely independent. It is a ventricular escape rhythm based on the wide and bizarre morphology of the QRS complexes and also based on the rate of the escape rhythm (38 bpm). A junctional escape rhythm typically has QRS complexes that are of normal morphology (tall, narrow and upright in lead II) with an escape rate of 40–60 bpm.

ii. In this Cocker Spaniel, a transvenous endocardial pacemaker was implanted as treatment for third-degree AV block.

iii. Pacemaker implantation is indicated in cases of symptomatic bradyarrhythmias including AV block (as in this case), sick sinus syndrome and persistent atrial standstill.

iv. The approach used to perform a transvenous endocardial pacemaker implantation is a cutdown to the external jugular vein. This allows cannulation of the jugular vein and access to the heart. Percutaneous access is less painful than the traditional surgical access.

v. The tip of a transvenous endocardial pacemaker is located in the apex of the right ventricle.

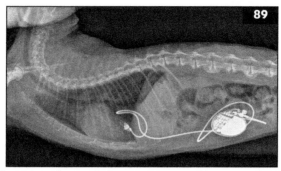

89 A lateral thoracic radiograph from a 17-year-old castrated, male Persian cat with the same diagnosis as **Case 88** is shown (**89**).

i. What treatment was performed in this case?

ii. What was the approach in this case?

iii. Where is the ideal location for placement of the lead on the heart?

iv. What do each of the letters in the five letter code represent?

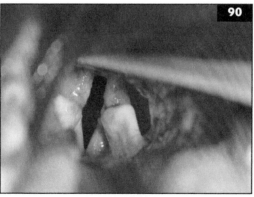

90 A 10-year-old spayed, female Labrador Retriever presents for dyspnea and an intraoral photograph was taken (**90**). The owners report that over the last 2 years, the dog's bark has changed, the dog has experienced intermittent increased respiratory effort and seems to scuff the hind feet with increasing frequency.

i. What is the suspected diagnosis? How will you confirm the diagnosis?

ii. What surgical procedures could be performed?

iii. Why is this dog scuffing the hind feet?

89i. This cat had an epicardial pacemaker implanted. This cat had an epicardial pacemaker rather than a transjugular endocardial pacemaker because of the small size of the cat's vasculature.

ii. In this case, a laparotomy with transdiaphragmatic approach was used. A transxiphoid approach could also be used (Nelson, 2012).

iii. Ideally, the epicardial pacemaker will be placed on the apex of the left ventricle.

iv. The letters in the five letter code each identify pacemaker function. The first letter indicates the chamber paced (O: none; A: atrium; V: ventricle; D: dual). The second letter indicates the chamber sensed (O: none; A: atrium; V: ventricle; D: dual). The third letter indicates the response to sensing (O: none; I: inhibited; T: triggered; D: dual). The fourth letter indicates the programmability/rate modulation (O: none; P: simple programmable; M: multiprogrammable antitachyarrhythmia; C: communicating; R: rate modulation). The fifth letter indicates antitachyarrhythmia functions (O: none; P: pacing; S: shock; D: dual).

90i. The suspected diagnosis is laryngeal paralysis. This disease process is often diagnosed in older large breed dogs (Labrador Retrievers are over-represented). The affected dogs often present with dyspnea, heat intolerance, change in bark and exercise intolerance. This diagnosis is confirmed with a sedated laryngeal exam. The animal should be in a light plane of anesthesia. Doxapram can be administered to elicit maximal respiratory effort during the laryngeal examination.

ii. Several surgical procedures are available for this condition. Unilateral arytenoid lateralization (by either cricoarytenoid lateralization or thyroarytenoid lateralization) is quite successful. Other options include ventriculocordectomy (ventral or transoral approach), partial laryngectomy, abductor muscle prosthesis, muscle-nerve transposition, modified castellated laryngofissure and permanent tracheostomy. Bilateral ventriculocordectomy performed through a ventral laryngotomy is reported to have a good outcome and minimal complications (Zikes, 2012). Transoral bilateral ventriculocordectomy results in stenosis of the rima glottidis, requiring a second surgery in over 10% of cases.

iii. Many older dogs with laryngeal paralysis are suspected to have a poly-neuropathy. Loss of conscious proprioception (scuffing feet) may be a clinical sign of polyneuropathy, as may laryngeal paralysis (Thieman, 2010). Esophageal dysfunction and the development of generalized neuropathy in older dogs with laryngeal paralysis are common, prompting the term 'geriatric onset laryngeal paralysis polyneuropathy' (GOLPP) syndrome (Stanley, 2010).

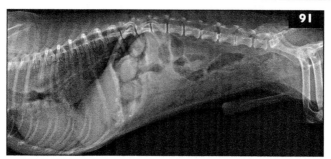

91 A 5-year-old Dachshund presents for a 1-week history of vomiting. On physical examination, there are no obvious abnormalities and no pain is elicited on abdominal palpation.
i. Identify abnormalities on this lateral radiograph (91). What bloodwork abnormalities would be expected for this patient when performing a CBC and serum biochemistry profile?
ii. What treatment options are possible for this patient?
iii. Regarding surgical treatment, what suture pattern(s) is/are recommended for closure of the gastric wall?

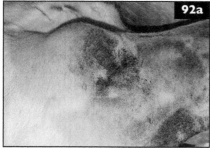

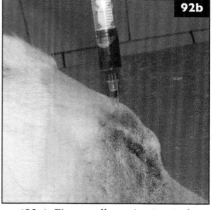

92 A 6–year-old female Central Asian Shepherd dog is admitted for further evaluation and treatment of a painful periorbital swelling, protrusion of the third eye lid and exopthalmos of the right eye (92a). Fine needle aspiration is done and a blood-stained and tenacious fluid compatible with saliva is obtained (92b).
i. What is your diagnosis?
ii. What are your differentials?
iii. How common is this condition and what treatment do you recommend?

91i. Multiple ovoid foreign bodies are present in the gastric lumen. Megaesophagus is present in the caudal thorax. Expected bloodwork abnormalities would include hemoconcentration and prerenal azotemia secondary to dehydration due to prolonged vomiting. Hypokalemia, hypernatremia or hyponatremia and hypochloremia may be present due to both dehydration and loss of gastric acid through vomiting. Acid–base status can vary from metabolic alkalosis (due to loss of hydrochloric acid in vomiting), to metabolic acidosis (due to loss of bicarbonate from duodenum).

ii. Endoscopy could be used to remove the oval foreign bodies (acorns). If unavailable, a gastrotomy could be performed to remove the foreign bodies. Gastric feeding tube placement could be considered due to the presence of megaesophagus. If no feeding tube is placed, the owner should be instructed to feed the patient in an elevated manner. Regardless of treatment option, sucralfate should be administered to treat any possible gastric ulcers. A proton pump inhibitor, such as omeprazole, or an acid (H2) blocker, such as famotidine, could be administered to prevent increased acid production and ulcer formation.

iii. Gastrotomy incisions should be closed in two layers. The first layer can either be an inverting pattern or, more commonly, a simple continuous appositional pattern. The second layer should be an inverting pattern, preferably with a Cushing or Lembert suture pattern. Since a Connell pattern passes into the gastric lumen, its use is discouraged if possible.

92i. This dog has a zygomatic sialocele.

ii. Differential diagnosis includes a zygomatic abscess associated with sialoadenitis or foreign body, space-occupying orbital lesions and zygomatic or oropharyngeal neoplasms.

iii. Zygomatic sialocele is a rare type of sialocele that requires zygomatic gland excision through a lateral orbitotomy. This is achieved by performing a skin and subcutaneous incision over the dorsal rim of the zygomatic arch. The orbital fascia and ligament are elevated dorsally. Partial zygomatic arch ostectomy or osteotomy is performed, allowing for a better visualization and exposure of the gland. The globe is retracted dorsally to expose periorbital fat and zygomatic gland (**92c**).

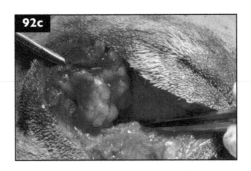

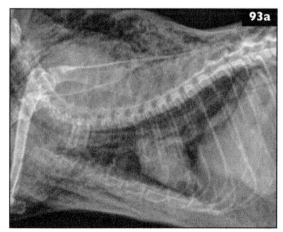

93 A 9-year-old neutered, male Himalayan cat presented with a 6-day history of progressive subcutaneous emphysema, originating around the head and neck. There was no history of trauma. Dental prophylaxis under general anesthesia had been performed 10 days previously.
i. List the radiographic abnormalities (93a).
ii. What is the likely diagnosis?
iii. How can this condition be definitively diagnosed?
iv. What are reported risk factors for this condition?
v. What is the recommended treatment?

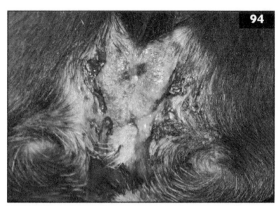

94 The perianal area of a neutered male Boston Terrier is shown (94).
i. What is your diagnosis and recommended surgical therapy?
ii. What are common postoperative complications associated with this procedure?

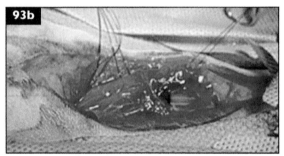

93i. There is marked subcutaneous emphysema within the soft tissues of the caudal cervical, thoracic and cranial abdominal regions, pneumomediastinum and a low-volume pneumo-thorax.

ii. Iatrogenic tracheal tear or tracheal necrosis secondary to endotracheal intubation for recent dental prophylaxis should be suspected, given the recent history.

iii. Endoscopic examination is reported to be the most useful modality for diagnosis and localization of the tear (Hardie, 1999; Mitchell, 2000). CT has also been reported to successfully delineate a tracheal tear in one cat (Bhandal, 2008).

iv. 70% of cats with iatrogenic tracheal tears were reported to have had recent dental prophylaxis (Mitchell, 2000). Factors contributing to the increased frequency of tracheal tears associated with this procedure may include the frequent alteration of head position, as well as over-inflation of the cuff to minimize aspiration of debris (Hardie, 1999).

v. Conservative therapy consisting of cage rest, sedation and supplemental oxygen was successful in 15/19 (79%) cats (Mitchell, 2000). Surgical exploration of the cervical region may be required if emphysema is progressive or results in severe respiratory distress (**93b**).

94i. The photograph shows a dog with bilateral ruptured anal sac abscesses. Surgical removal of both anal sacs is recommended. This surgery can be performed in one procedure or as staged procedures. Many dogs with rupture of the anal sac abscess require antibiotic treatment and flushing of the duct and wound prior to surgical treatment, as in this case. Preoperative medical management may reduce inflammation and facilitate surgical removal. Occasionally, anal sac impaction and/or abscessation can occur secondary to a neoplastic process. Tissues removed during surgery should be submitted for histopathology.

ii. Overall, the rate of complications associated with anal sacculectomy is low. Fecal incontinence, chronic draining tracts, tenesmus and stricture formation are all potential complications. Fecal incontinence typically occurs subsequent to damage to the external anal sphincter or caudal rectal nerve during dissection. If damage is unilateral, fecal incontinence may be temporary until reinnervation from the contralateral side occurs.

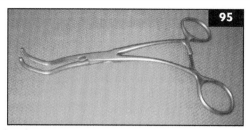

95 A 7 year-old Labrador Retriever presents for polyuria and polydipsia. Bloodwork and thoracic radiographs were unremarkable but an enlarged right adrenal gland was noted on abdominal ultrasound. A CT scan reveals a 5 cm adrenal mass that appears to invade the caudal vena cava.

i. What are your options for surgical removal from the vena cava? What is the mortality rate associated with adrenalectomy and how does tumoral invasion of the vena cava affect prognosis?

ii. What vascular clamp can be used to assist with surgical removal (95)? If complete occlusion of the caudal vena cava is necessary, what can be applied to occlude blood flow temporarily but completely? For what duration of time can flow through the caudal vena cava be completely occluded?

iii. What are the three layers of blood vessel walls? What is the principal cell type of each wall layer? What suture pattern is generally recommended for vessel wall closure and what type of suture is preferred?

96 A 10-year-old mixed breed dog presents for evaluation. Several months ago, the dog had an episode and was hospitalized. During that time, the dog's liver enzyme activities were elevated but returned to normal 2 weeks later. One month ago, the dog's activity level and appetite decreased. On bloodwork, the liver enzyme activities are decreased. The serum levels of cholesterol, albumin and BUN are all decreased. An ammonia level is tested and is elevated. You perform an abdominal exploratory (96).

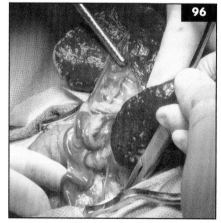

i. What is your diagnosis?

ii. What less invasive techniques could have been utilized to make this diagnosis?

95i. A venotomy of the caudal vena cava can be performed to remove the tumor thrombus from the vena cava. Reported mortality rates associated with adrenalectomy range from 15% to 25%. In one study, invasion of the caudal vena cava, particularly if the tumor thrombus extends beyond the hepatic hilus, is associated with a higher postoperative mortality rate. Invasion of the vena cava did not affect long-term prognosis (Barrera, 2013).

ii. Satinsky forceps can be placed tangentially to the vena cava to allow partial occlusion. The area that had undergone venotomy can be included within the clamp to facilitate closure while the remainder of the vena cava is patent. Complete occlusion of the vena cava can be achieved with Rumel tourniquets. A Rumel tourniquet comprises umbilical tape, which is placed around the vessel to be occluded, and a short piece of tubing (such as a red rubber catheter) that can be placed over the ends of the umbilical tape and pulled down into the vessel to compress it. A hemostat is placed on the tubing to hold the tourniquet in place. Debate exists over the recommended duration of vena cava occlusion. A general recommendation is to limit occlusion to as short a time as possible and no more than 20–30 minutes.

iii. The outer layer of the vessel is the adventitia, which is made up of connective tissue and the associated blood supply to the wall of the blood vessel itself. Care is taken to not disrupt excessive portions of the adventitia. The middle layer, or media, is the muscular layer containing smooth muscle and elastin. The inner layer, or intima, is made up of endothelial cells. A simple continuous line is commonly used for vascular surgery; polypropylene is preferred (sizes 4-0 to 7-0, depending on the vessel) with suture passing full thickness through all three layers.

96i. This dog appears to have multiple acquired portosystemic shunts. Multiple tortuous vessels can be seen extending through this dog's abdomen. In this dog, the veins join the renal vein and the caudal vena cava in the area of the kidneys. This distribution of multiple acquired portosystemic shunts is typical but shunts may connect to other systemic vessels. Liver biopsies are performed.

ii. Less invasive techniques that can be used to diagnose portosystemic shunts include: abdominal ultrasound, nuclear scintigraphy (transcolonic or transsplenic), CT angiography and MRI angiography. Laparoscopic evaluation of this dog may have provided visualization of the multiple acquired portosystemic shunts. Portovenography is another imaging modality but requires a laparotomy to be performed and is also considered an invasive procedure.

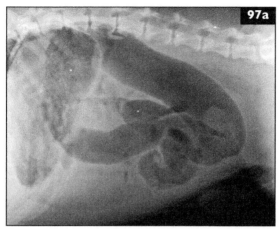

97 A radiograph of a 4-year-old Mastiff is shown (97a). The dog presented for acute onset abdominal pain with no history of trauma. On examination, the dog was laterally recumbent with signs of hypovolemic shock. The abdomen was mildly enlarged. Pain was elicited on palpation of the abdomen. The dog underwent exploratory laparotomy and was diagnosed with a colonic torsion.
i. What predisposing factors are associated with colonic torsion?
ii. What is the difference between intestinal torsion and intestinal volvulus?
iii. What prognosis is associated with colonic torsion?
iv. What treatment should be performed?

98 An 8-year-old spayed, female mixed breed dog presents with presence of a septic abdominal effusion. At the time of surgery, a perforated duodenal ulcer is identified along with severe thickening of the pyloric antrum. Multiple erosions and ulcers are noted throughout the gastric mucosa. The owner reports a chronic history of vomiting, weight loss, anorexia and intermittent diarrhea.
i. What are the differential diagnoses for the cause of gastroduodenal ulcerations in the dog?
ii. Where is gastrin produced in the dog? What is the most common location for gastrinoma formation in the dog?

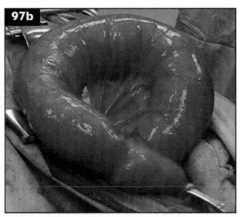

97i. A previously performed gastropexy or previous treatment of gastric dilatation volvulus may increase the chance of colonic torsion. Rupture of the gastroduodenal ligament or previously formed intestinal adhesions may also increase the risk of colonic torsion. Although colonic torsion is a rare condition, studies suggest that large breed dogs are predisposed (Gagnon, 2013).

ii. Intestinal torsion describes the twisting of a segment of intestine around the longitudinal axis. Intestinal volvulus describes rotation of the intestines around the mesenteric root.

iii. The mortality associated with intestinal volvulus is high. Likewise, the mortality rate associated with colonic torsion is believed to be high. With early surgical intervention, the prognosis may be improved. In one report, 5/5 dogs with early surgical intervention had a successful outcome (Gagnon, 2013).

iv. The dog should undergo exploratory surgery (**97b**). At the time of surgery, devitalized tissue should be resected. A left lateral body wall colopexy should be performed.

98i. Gastroduodenal ulcerations occur in association with a number of causes/ disease processes in the dog which include: administration of non-steroidal anti-inflammatories, administration of steroidal anti-inflammatories, hypoadreno-corticism, renal dysfunction/uremia, hepatic disease, mastocytosis, disseminated intravascular coagulation, hypergastrinemia/gastrinoma, APUDomas (endocrine tumor arising from an APUD cell; also known as neuroendocrine gastroentero-pancreatic tumor), gastritis, leiomyoma/leiomyosarcoma, adenocarcinoma, lymphoma, shock/hypotension/hypoperfusion, sepsis, stress and induced by exercise (this is uncommonly diagnosed in sled dogs).

ii. In dogs, gastrin is primarily secreted from G cells located in the gastric antrum and duodenum. Pancreatic islet cells (delta cells) are a site of production of gastrin in fetal and neonatal animals and are the most common site of gastrinoma formation.

99 Regarding the dog in **Case 98**, list at least three medical therapies that can palliate clinical signs that occur as a consequence of hypergastrinemia. Provide drug classes and a brief description of mechanism of action and/or reason for use of each drug class.

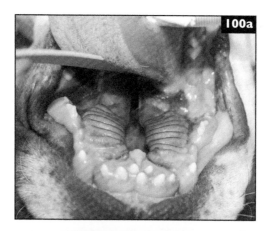

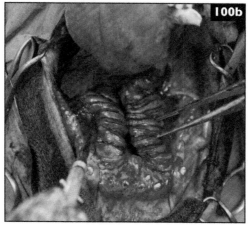

100 Preoperative and intraoperative photographs are shown (**100a, b**).
i. What congenital abnormality is being repaired in this dog?
ii. What procedure is being performed?
iii. At what age should this procedure be performed?

99 1. Histamine (H2) receptor antagonists (cimetidine, ranitidine, famotidine): block H2 receptors on parietal cells in the stomach to decrease hydrochloric acid production. Gastrin is a potent stimulator of gastric acid secretion. Blocking H2 receptors will decrease gastric acid secretion, which is desirable in this dog.

2. H^+/K^+ adenosine triphosphatase (ATPase) inhibitors/proton pump inhibitors (omeprazole, lansoprazole, pantoprazole, esomeprazole, rabeprazole): block the H^+/K^+ ATPase pump which is the final step in acid secretion and binding is irreversible. Again, this drug class will decrease the secretion of acid.

3. Diffusion barriers (sucralfate): sucralfate dissociates in the acidic environment of the stomach into aluminum hydroxide and sucrose octasulfate. Sucrose octasulfate undergoes polymerization and has a strong negative charge that binds to the positively charged proteins in the base of ulcers or erosions, and forms a barrier that protects the ulcer from further damage. Sucralfate also stimulates production of prostaglandins and growth factors that protect the gastric mucosa.

4. Synthetic prostaglandins (misoprostol): this class both inhibits acid production (minimal decrease in activity of H^+/K^+ ATPase) and protects gastric mucosa by increasing bicarbonate secretion and mucus production and enhancing mucosal blood flow.

5. Somatostatin analogs (octreotide): somatostatin inhibits gastrin and hydrogen ion secretion in gastrinomas and in gastric parietal cells. This drug class directly inhibits the excessively produced gastrin to prevent over-secretion of acid.

100i. This dog has a congenital cleft of the secondary palate. The secondary palate consists of the hard and soft palates. The primary palate includes the lip and premaxilla (which were normal in this dog).

ii. This palatoplasty is being performed by a bipedical advancement technique. The mucoperiosteum of the palate is incised along the cleft and along the lingual surface of the teeth. The mucoperiosteum is carefully elevated, protecting the major palatine vessels. The bipedical flap is then advanced axially and sutured to the cut surface of the contralateral side of the cleft. In this case, two flaps were required to provide tension release and coverage of the cleft. Two flaps are frequently required if the cleft is $\geq 25\%$ of the width of the palate. In this case, the bipedical flaps were sutured with simple interrupted sutures alternating with vertical mattress sutures. The vertical mattress sutures provide some eversion, allowing tissue planes to align and heal.

iii. This procedure should be performed when the pet is older than 8 weeks of age. Waiting until after 4–5 months of age may be ideal as the collagen content of the tissues increases with age and has better holding strength. Additionally, the relative width of the defect decreases in relation to the amount of palatal tissues present, providing a greater amount of mucosa to close the defect.

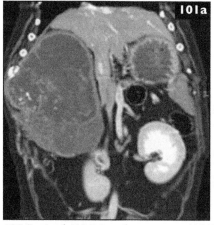
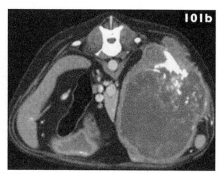

101 Sagittal (**101a**) and transverse (**101b**) CT images of a 7-year-old Weimaraner are presented.
i. Describe the CT findings.
ii. What are the three most common primary tumors in this location?
iii. What are options for closure of the defect created?
iv. What are possible postoperative complications related to this surgical procedure?

102 A 5-year-old spayed, female Maltese dog presents for a draining tract located beneath the right eye. The dog was previously treated with oral antibiotics. The draining tract healed during antibiotic administration and recurred at the discontinuation of the antibiotics.
i. What is the diagnosis and potential causes?
ii. What tests might be performed in order to confirm a diagnosis?
iii. What treatment should be performed?

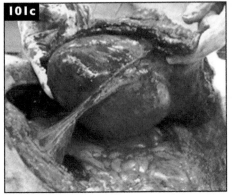

101i. Arising from the right caudal body wall there is a large, heterogenous, encapsulated, cavitated mass. Irregular periosteal new bone formation is present in the ribs the mass is in contact with. The mass disrupts the body wall, resulting in a component of the mass that is within the abdomen and a component of the mass that expands dorsolateral from the body wall. There is moderate displacement of the abdominal organs and vessels attributed to mass effect. The mass remains caudal to the diaphram (101c) but extends cranially within the abdomen and extends caudally along the dorsal aspect of body wall.

ii. Osteosarcoma, chondrosarcoma and hemangiosarcoma are the most common primary tumors in this location.

iii. Autogenous reconstruction including latissimus dorsi or deep pectoral muscle flaps, prosthetic reconstruction including mesh implants, such as Marlex, or composite reconstruction which is a combination of autogenous and prosthetic techniques. Advancement of the diaphragm can reduce the size of the thoracic defect when the tumor is located in the caudal thorax.

iv. Possible complications following chest wall resection include pleural effusion, seroma, surgical site infection, muscular flap necrosis from vascular compromise and respiratory failure.

102i. This dog has a tooth root abscess of the maxillary fourth premolar which has opened dorsally and is draining from the skin just ventral to the eye. Tooth root abscesses in this location can be seen as localized swelling, with or without a draining tract, either in the caudodorsal aspect of the muzzle or ventral to the eye (as in this dog). Alternatively, a draining tract may be seen at the mucogingival junction or may manifest itself as nasal discharge. Potential causes include fracture of the tooth with exposed pulp, extension of a periodontal pocket or concussive disease to the root.

ii. An oral examination should be performed to determine if fractured teeth are present or to identify devitalized or discolored teeth. Dental radiographs or CT scan of the head can be performed to confirm the diagnosis of tooth root abscess and identify which tooth is diseased.

iii. Treatment options include tooth extraction or root canal. Concurrent antibiotic therapy is appropriate and should cover anaerobic and gram-positive aerobic bacteria.

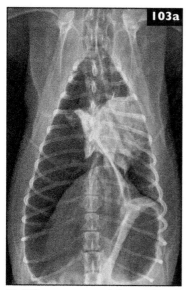

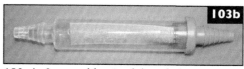

103 A 3-year-old mixed breed dog presents for retching and hypersalivation. Radiographs are taken and an esophageal foreign body (FB) is present. You have decided to perform esophagoscopy to attempt removal of the FB and evaluate the esophagus for perforation in order to determine the surgical approach needed. The dog is placed under general anesthesia and you begin insufflation for the esophagoscopy. Ventilation of the dog becomes difficult and you take this radiograph (103a). You decide to place a thoracic drain. You attach this device to the thoracic drain (103b).
i. What is this device?
ii. What is its function?
iii. What are potential complications associated with use of this device?

104 An image of the perineum of a 9-month-old male Greyhound with an acute onset of tenesmus is shown (104a).
i. List two differentials for the condition shown.
ii. How would you differentiate between the two conditions?
iii. What would be your treatment(s) for the two conditions?
iv. How might you prevent recurrence of the described conditions?

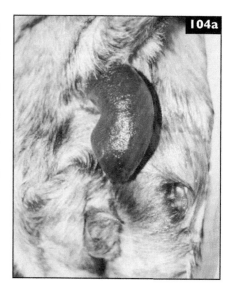

Answers: 103, 104

103i. This is a Heimlich valve (also known as a flutter valve).

ii. The Heimlich valve is a device that provides continuous drainage of the thoracic cavity. The Heimlich valve is a one-way valve that uses the animal's breath to displace air or fluid through the valve. This device can provide early mobility or easy transportation to the patient as it does not require the application of negative pressure, nor does it require that a thoracic drain be clamped.

iii. Potential complications associated with use of the Heimlich valve include failure of the valve diaphragm preventing drainage from the thorax and open pneumothorax from damage to the valve itself. Inappropriate use of the valve can lead to tension pneumothorax.

104i. Rectal prolapse or prolapsed intussusception.

ii. Insertion of a probe alongside the prolapsed tissue will distinguish between rectal prolapse and prolapsed intussusception. In this case, an endoscope has been passed alongside the prolapsed tissue for a distance of 15 cm (**104b**). The diagnosis is therefore a prolapsed intussusception.

iii. With both conditions, manual reduction can be attempted if the tissue is viable. In the case of rectal prolapse, reduction of healthy prolapsed tissue and temporary placement of an anal purse string suture can be performed. In rectal prolapse, if non-viable tissue is present, amputation of non-viable tissue should be performed. In cases with prolapsed intussusception, exploratory laparotomy must also be performed with reduction and or resection and anastomosis of the intussusception.

iv. With simple rectal prolapse, colopexy is often effective to prevent recurrence. Enteropexy might be considered for prevention of prolapsed intussusception, but the efficacy of this procedure is controversial.

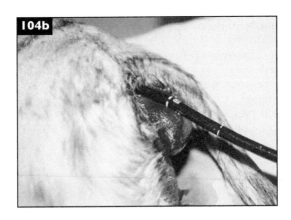

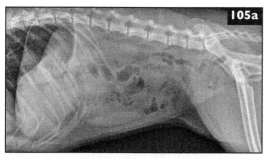
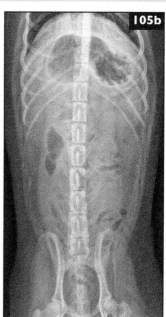
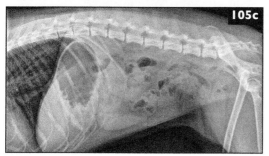

105 A 3-year-old spayed, female mixed breed dog presents for acute onset of vomiting of 24 hours duration. A three view radiographic study of the abdomen is shown (**105a–c**).

i. Describe your radiographic findings and your presumptive diagnosis.

ii. Describe your surgical approach and intervention.

iii. Name a potential pre-/perioperative complication.

iv. What are risk factors that increase the risk for postoperative intestinal dehiscence?

106 What are three applications for cyanoacrylates in veterinary medicine?

105i. There are multiple comma/geometrically-shaped gas opacities in the small bowel in the mid-abdomen as would occur with plicated bowel. The descending duodenum is displaced on the ventrodorsal view. Air does not fill the pylorus on the left lateral view. These findings are all consistent with a linear foreign body (FB), potentially anchored in the stomach. The serosal detail remains good with no indication of perforation or peritonitis at this time.

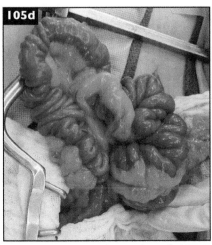

ii. This dog needs an abdominal exploratory surgery. If the FB extends from the pylorus into the proximal small intestine, the first approach would be to see if the entire FB can be removed via a gastrotomy. If not, then the FB is transected intraluminally in the stomach, the gastric portion of the FB is removed, and the remaining portions removed through enterotomies. Alternatively, once the linear FB is transected, the free end of the aboral FB can be sutured to a red rubber catheter. The catheter can be milked through the intestines, removing the foreign material as the catheter is moved aborally. This technique decreases or eliminates the need for multiple enterotomies but can be time consuming and difficult to perform.

iii. The restrictive nature of a linear FB and the intestinal plication places this patient at high risk for intestinal perforation (**105d**).

iv. Risk factors for intestinal dehiscence include preoperative septic peritonitis, hypoproteinemia, hypoalbuminemia and intraoperative hypotension (Grimes, 2011).

106 The most common applications of cyanoacrylate glue are dermal and ocular. When the liquid cyanoacrylate is exposed to an anion (such as those found in water or blood), the liquid glue polymerizes and bonds tissues. Correct application of cyanoacrylate is important. Tissue edges should be apposed and glue should be placed on the wound to bond the tissues but should not be allowed within the wound. Recently, cyanoacrylates have been reported for use in percutaneous embolization of vascular anomalies such as arteriovenous malformations. Embolization of the thoracic duct with cyanoacrylate glue has been reported to treat chylothorax (Weisse, 2008).

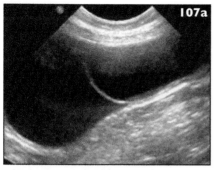 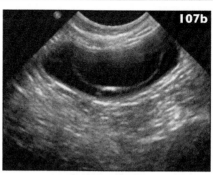

107 An 8-month-old intact, female mixed breed dog presents for further evaluation of chronic urinary tract infections, stranguria, pollakiuria and intermittent urinary incontinence. Sagittal and transverse sonographic images of the urinary bladder are provided (**107a, b**).
i. Describe the ultrasonographic findings. What is the diagnosis?
ii. What is the pathophysiology of this condition?
iii. Discuss treatment options.

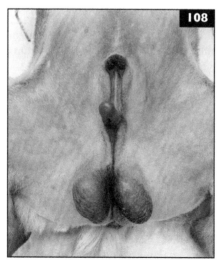

108 Consider the dog in photograph **108**.
i. What is your diagnosis?
ii. In what breed of dog is this anomaly most prevalent?
iii. Where can the external urethral orifice be located with this anomaly?
iv. What treatment should be recommended?

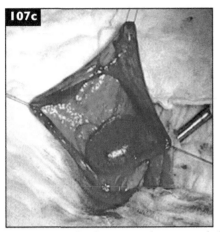

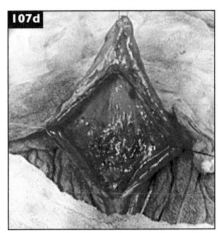

107i. Towards the trigonal region of the urinary bladder a large, thin-walled, anechoic, fluid-filled structure is present which may be associated with the ureteral papilla. Diagnosis is most likely an orthotopic or intravesicular ureterocele.

ii. Ureteroceles are thought to occur as a result of dysembryogenesis. Proposed mechanisms are the failure of Chwalle's membrane to regress, abnormalities with fusion of the metanephric duct and urogenital sinus and alterations within the connective tissue and muscle of the distal ureter. Chwalle's membrane normally separates the common excretory duct and the ureter. Ureteroceles are described as being orthotopic or intravesicular if the ureterocele is within the urinary bladder and the ureteral opening is located in a normal anatomical position. Ectopic ureteroceles are found concurrently with ureteral ectopia and are located within the urethra and associated with urinary incontinence.

iii. For orthotopic ureteroceles, urethral obstruction, stranguria and pollakiuria is likely a result of the dilated ureterocele (**107c**). For those cases, ureterocelectomy without revision of the ureteral opening is recommended (**107d**). For ectopic ureteroceles, ureterocelectomy along with neoureterocystostomy is indicated, depending on clinical signs.

108i. This dog has hypospadias and incomplete preputial fusion. Hypospadias is the most common congenital abnormality of the male external genitalia. This anomaly occurs due to incomplete fusion of the urogenital folds and incomplete formation of the penile urethra.

ii. This congenital abnormality occurs most commonly in the Boston Terrier.

iii. In hypospadias, the external urethral orifice can be present in glandular, penile, scrotal, perineal and anal locations.

iv. Orchidectomy with removal of preputial and penile remnants and enlargement of scrotal or perineal urethral orifice (scrotal or perineal urethrostomy) may be performed if necessary. Some dogs with hypospadias are not clinical and do not require treatment.

109 A 10-year-old castrated, male mixed breed dog presents for a chole-cystectomy (109). On blood work, ALP, ALT and total bilirubin are elevated. No other abnormalities are found. The dog was premedicated with glycopyrrolate and methadone, and anesthesia was induced with propofol. The dog is being maintained under anesthesia with sevoflurane delivery in 100% oxygen and a remifentanil CRI. The dog has been under general anesthesia for 30

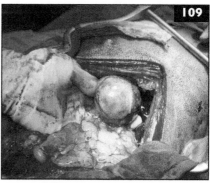

minutes and all the parameters are within normal limits. Once dissection of the gall bladder has taken place, a sudden decrease in end-tidal (Et) CO_2 from 35 mmHg to 22 mmHg occurs. The dog's heart rate decreases from 98 bpm to 35 bpm, and continues to drop. You see a flat line in the arterial wave pressure, ECG and capnograph.

i. What is happening and what should you do?
ii. What should you do immediately according to the Reassessment Campaign on Veterinary Resuscitation (RECOVER) clinical guidelines?
iii. Why are large amounts of fluids not recommended if the patient is euvolemic?

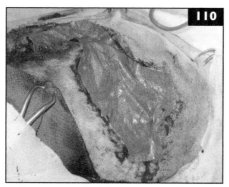

110 A wound dressing impregnated with nanocrystaline silver is shown (110).
i. For what purpose is silver impregnated in the bandage material?
ii. How does the silver perform its role?

109i. The monitoring equipment is indicating the patient is suffering a cardiorespiratory arrest. You should confirm your suspicion **quickly** by checking a pulse and for equipment malfunction.

ii. Taking into consideration the owner's decision to resuscitate or not, the first action is to turn off the inhalants and any analgesic being administered to the patient and begin basic life support. Since the dog is already intubated the airway patency is secured and the dog is receiving high inspiratory fraction of oxygen (FiO_2 = 100%), ventilator (manual or mechanical) support (10–24 breaths per minute) may be started. Cardiac massage (80–120 compressions/minute) should begin immediately. For this particular case, internal massage will be applied since the abdominal cavity is open, allowing the heart to be reached through the diaphragm.

Advanced life support with support of circulation and administration of drugs is simultaneously initiated. Atropine (0.04 mg/kg IV) should be administered quickly to reduce vagal tone. Vasopressors, such as epinephrine (0.01 mg/kg low dose) or vasopressin (0.8 U/kg IV), should be used to increase peripheral vascular resistance to redirect blood volume to the central circulation, to perfuse the myocardium and the brain. Uninterrupted cycles (2 minutes) of cardiac massage and ventilation should be established and after those cycles quickly assess for the return of spontaneous circulation, or for the need of antiarrhythmic drugs or defibrillation. High doses of epinephrine (0.1 mg/kg iv) may be considered if the patient is not responding to the low dose. Repeated doses of drugs can be administered every 3–5 minutes as needed. In this naloxone (0.002–0.02 mg/kg IV) should be administered to reverse previously administered opioids.

iii. Large amounts of fluid administered to an euvolemic patient result in increased right atrial pressure, impaired coronary perfusion and further compromises the myocardium.

110i. Silver has pronounced antibacterial activity against Gram-positive and Gram-negative bacteria. The antimicrobial activity of silver includes many resistant bacteria such as methicillin-resistant strains. Silver is also effective against some strains of yeast and fung**i.**

ii. Silver must be present in its ionized form to function as an antimicrobial. The silver ions are hypothesized to inhibit bacterial protein synthesis and denature bacterial DNA.

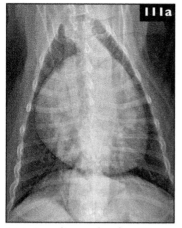

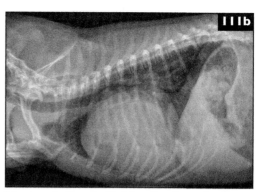

111 A radiograph of a 10-year-old spayed, female Golden Retriever is shown (**111a, b**). The dog presented for collapse. On physical examination, muffled heart sounds were detected and thoracic radiography was performed.
i. What procedure(s) should be performed?
ii. What are differential diagnoses?

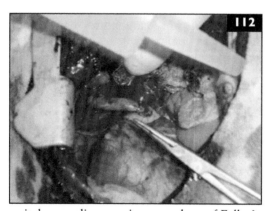

112 i. What congenital anomalies constitute tetralogy of Fallot?
ii. What are the pathophysiologic consequences of tetralogy of Fallot?
iii. Pictured is a completed surgical procedure performed on a dog with tetralogy of Fallot (**112**). The dog's head is to the left and the thoracic organs are visible through the lateral intercostal thoracotomy approach. What procedure has been performed?

111i. Interpretation of the radiograph reveals pericardial effusion. A pericardiocentesis should be performed. This procedure is the best emergency treatment of cardiac tamponade. The fluid removed from the pericardial sac should be collected. The fluid may be hemorrhagic in appearance but should not clot after removal. If the blood does clot, the heart may have been punctured and blood may have been removed instead of effusion. The fluid removed from the pericardium should be submitted for cytologic evaluation and culture. In addition to thoracic radiographs and pericardiocentesis, echocardiography should be performed. Echocardiography may aid in the diagnosis of cardiac neoplasia, constrictive pericarditis and pericardial cysts. Bloodwork including a CBC, serum chemistry panel and coagulation panel should be performed.

ii. Differential diagnoses will depend on clinical pathologic characteristics of the fluid. Transudates may occur due to heart failure, peritoneal–pericardial diaphragmatic hernia, hypoalbuminemia and vasculitis. Exudates may occur secondary to pericarditis (infectious/non-infectious). Hemorrhagic effusion may occur secondary to trauma, cardiac neoplasia, ruptured right atrium, coagulopathy or idiopathic. In this dog, neoplasia would be a viable differential diagnosis. Hemangiosarcoma of the right atrium is the most common cardiac neoplasm. The tumor may be multicentric, involving the spleen, liver or elsewhere. An abdominal work-up including ultrasound should be recommended as 29% of dogs with cardiac hemangiosarcoma have a concurrent splenic hemangiosarcoma, and 42% of dogs with cardiac hemangiosarcoma have metastasis to another site (Boston, 2011).

112i. Tetralogy of Fallot consists of four abnormalities: ventricular septal defect, dextrapositioned over-riding aorta, pulmonic stenosis and right ventricular hypertrophy.

ii. Tetralogy of Fallot can result in increased right sided ventricular pressure, right to left circulatory shunting and bypass of the pulmonary circulation. This results in chronic systemic hypoxemia, and subsequent polycythemia. Clinical results include cyanosis and exercise intolerance.

iii. A modified Blalock–Taussig shunt has been created. This technique utilizes an autogenous jugular venograft to create a left to right shunt through anastomosis of the left subclavian artery (systemic circulation) to the pulmonary artery (pulmonary circulation). Several systemic to pulmonary shunts have been described including Blalock–Taussig, Potts (aorticopulmonary anastomosis), Waterson (aorta to right pulmonary artery anastomosis), and Glenn (venocaval to pulmonary artery anastomosis). Systemic to pulmonary shunts are considered palliative procedures, and definitive open correction for tetralogy of Fallot can be undertaken in dogs with the aid of cardiopulmonary bypass.

113 A 9-year-old castrated, male Labrador Retriever presents for evaluation of generalized weakness, ataxia and seizures. CBC and biochemistry were performed and revealed a blood glucose level of 42 mg/dL (reference range 70–138 mg/dL). All other values were within normal limits.
i. What are your differential diagnoses?
ii. After further evaluation, insulinoma is your primary differential. What is the most common location(s) of insulinoma?
iii. What are the long-term treatment options for insulinoma?
iv. What should be considered when treating an acute hypoglycemic event in a patient with an insulinoma?

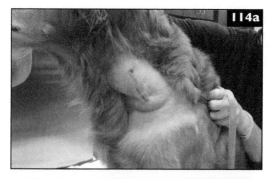

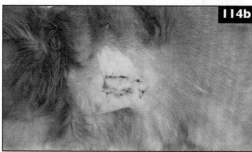

114 A 5-year-old Golden Retriever is shown, 3 days postoperatively following a sarcoma removal from the neck (**114a, b**).
i. Identify this postoperative complication.
ii. What is the preferred treatment option for this complication? If the preferred treatment option fails, what other more invasive treatment option could be performed?
iii. What major complication can occur with the more invasive treatment option and what can be done to prevent this complication?

113i. The primary differential diagnoses for hypoglycemia can be divided into three categories: (1) an oversecretion of insulin or insulin-like factors; (2) diminished glucose production; and (3) increased glucose consumption. Increased insulin secretion is associated with insulinoma, extrapancreatic tumor and islet cell hyperplasia. Decreased production of glucose can be associated with hepatic dysfunction, hypoadrenocorticism, glycogen storage disease, neonates, prolonged and severe fasting/malnutrition, hypopituitarism, growth hormone deficiency, toy breeds and occasionally pregnancy. Excessive consumption of glucose is associated with sepsis and extreme exertion (e.g. 'hunting dog hypoglycemia'). Other less common causes of hypoglycemia are drug related and spurious causes.

ii. The majority of insulinomas occur as a solitary pancreatic nodule affecting the right or left limb of the pancreas. The body of the pancreas is uncommonly involved.

iii. Partial pancreatectomy with surgical removal of gross metastatic disease identified at the time of surgery is the treatment of choice. Medical therapies are ideally used in conjunction with surgery and may include: dietary modification (diet high in protein, fat and complex carbohydrates fed in small frequent meals), corticosteroids, diazoxide, synthetic somatostatin and streptozocin.

iv. In the event of an emergent hypoglycemic event, intravenous dextrose (administered as a bolus and followed by a continuous rate infusion) is often utilized. This should be administered with caution as dextrose can stimulate further secretion of insulin and may worsen hypoglycemia.

114i. This dog has a seroma. Seromas usually result from failure to close dead space. Closure for this tumor was made especially difficult because of the tumor's location over the jugular vein.

ii. Warm packing with restricted activity is the preferred treatment option for a seroma. Most seromas will resolve with this treatment alone. If the seroma is too large or warm packing does not yield positive results, drainage of the seroma (with cytology and culture if warranted) can be performed. Prior to drainage, the area should be clipped and undergo sterile preparation. Following drainage, placement of tacking sutures should be performed. Drainage alone without tacking sutures will often result in recurrence of the seroma.

iii. Infection of the seroma and/or the seroma becoming an abscess are both serious concerns if the seroma is to be drained. Surgical preparation of the site should be performed prior to aspiration of the fluid to minimize the risk of infection. Further, drainage of the seroma should only be used as a last resort.

115 Two lateral thoracic radiographs are shown (**115a, b**).
i. What is the disorder that both patients suffer from?
ii. How is this diagnosed and severity of disease determined?

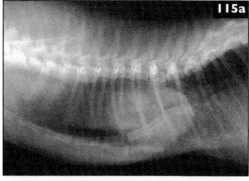

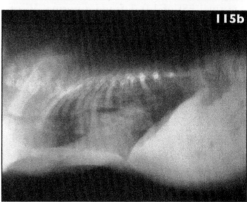

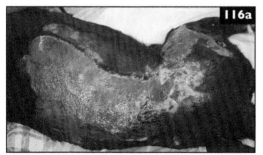

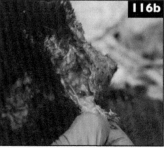

116 A 3-year-old Labrador mix was in a vehicle accident with the owners and suffered burns as a consequence (**116a, b**).
i. What is the classification of this burn injury?
ii. What are the zones of injury following a burn?

115i. Both of these animals have pectus excavatum. Pectus excavatum is a disorder in which the sternum and costal cartilages are abnormally formed. Animals with this disorder have a flattened thoracic cavity and concavity of the ventral thorax.
ii. Pectus excavatum is diagnosed by palpation or radiographs and severity is determined by measuring the fronto-sagittal index (FSI) or the vertebral index(VI) on lateral thoracic radiographs. The FSI is a ratio of the width of the chest at the 10th vertebral body to the dorsoventral measurement from the ventral surface of the 10th vertebra to the sternum. The VI is the ratio of the dorsoventral measurement of the dorsal surface of the vertebral body to the sternum to the dorsoventral measurement of the vertebral body itself. Several ranges have been established for different dog types as well as cats. Non-brachycephalic dogs have a normal FSI of 0.8–1.4 and a normal VI of 11.8–19.6. Brachycephalic dogs have a normal FSI of 1.0–1.5 and a normal VI of 12.5–16.5. Cats have a normal FSI of 0.7–1.3 and a normal VI of 12.6–18.8. The severity of clinical signs associated with the sternal deformity has not been correlated with FSI or VI.

116i. This dog has a combination of partial thickness (**116a**) and full thickness (**116b**) burns. Partial thickness burns are classified as first- and second-degree burns. First-degree burns are superficial, affecting only the epidermis. Second-degree burns extend into the dermis. Third-degree burns are full thickness burns. Third-degree burns extend through the skin and into the subcutaneous tissue. In this picture (**116b**), the burned skin is being removed (full thickness) to reveal granulation tissue forming underneath. The majority of this dog's wounds are second-degree and third-degree burns.
ii. The zones of injury include the zone of coagulation (also known as the zone of necrosis or zone of destruction), the zone of stasis and the zone of hyperemia. The zone of coagulation is the area of tissue that received the greatest damage. This tissue is no longer viable and will slough. The zone of stasis is the next area and this tissue experiences decreased perfusion. The vessels become narrowed because of tissue edema and the proteins in the area are damaged from heat. The tissues in the zone of stasis may survive but may undergo necrosis. The zone of hyperemia is an area of inflammation; the tissue in this zone is viable.

117 An 8-year-old intact male dog presents for decreased appetite, lethargy and penile discharge. On digital rectal examination, the prostate is enlarged. Pain is elicited on palpation of the prostate.
i. What diagnostic investigations should be performed?
ii. You suspect prostatitis. What bacteria are most likely causing bacterial prostatitis and what treatment is appropriate to administer?

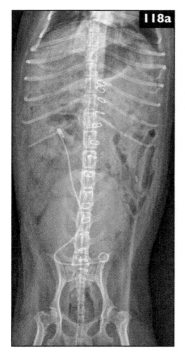

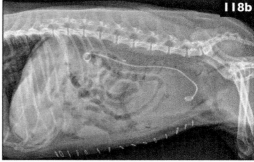

118 Postoperative radiographs of a dog that has undergone a procedure are shown (**118a, b**).
i. What implant has been placed in the dog?
ii. What are the indications for placement of this implant and what benefit does it provide?
iii. At what anatomic locations should this implant begin and terminate?

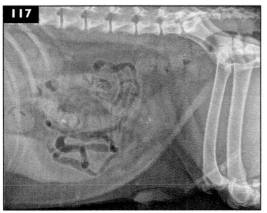

117i. Most prostatic disease causes enlargement of the prostate and this finding is not specific to a particular disease process. A CBC, serum chemistry and urinalysis (with urine culture) should be performed. A *Brucella canis* titer and abdominal radiographs should be performed. The radiographs may indicate an enlarged prostate (as in this case; [117]). Mineralization may be seen in the prostate. Mineralization is indicative of neoplasia in neutered males, but is not as specific in intact dogs. Abdominal ultrasound will provide more information. Ultrasonography should be helpful in the diagnosis of prostatitis, benign prostatic hypertrophy, abscessation, prostatic cysts or neoplasia. Ultrasonographic appearance in combination with ultrasound guided fine needle aspirates may provide a diagnosis.

ii. The most common organism in prostatitis infections is *Escherichia coli*. Other common bacteria include *Staphylococcus* species, *Proteus mirabilis*, *Klebsiella* species, *Mycoplasma* species and *Pseudomonas* species. Treatment of prostatitis should include the recommendation of castration. Castration provides involution of hyperplastic glands and decreased prostatic secretory function. Antibiotic therapy is ideally based on culture and sensitivity testing. The blood–lipid barrier in the normal prostate restricts antibiotic penetration of the prostate. In the inflamed prostate, antibiotics likely diffuse well into the tissue. Antibiotics that are known to have good prostate penetration include enroflaxacin, marbofloxacin, trimethoprim-sulfa and chloramphenicol.

118i. This dog has a ureteral stent (double-pigtail stent). This is a multifenestrated catheter with a pigtail loop on each end.

ii. This implant can be placed in dogs and cats for a variety of reasons, in the hope of maintaining urine flow from the renal pelvis to the urinary bladder. In dogs and cats, the implant has been described to relieve or prevent urinary obstruction due to trigonal urothelial carcinoma (Berent, 2011), ureteroliths, stone migration following extracorporeal shock-wave lithotripsy and ureteral stricture. Ureteral stents have many benefits including immediate decompression of the renal pelvis, passive ureteral dilation for urine and stone passage and prevention of stricture.

iii. The proximal portion of this implant is a pigtail loop that is curled in the renal pelvis. The shaft of the catheter is placed within the ureter and the distal pigtail loop is curled within the urinary bladder.

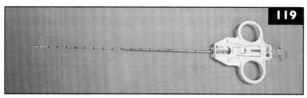

119 A 9-year-old spayed, female dog presents for further evaluation of proteinuria. The patient has been referred for renal biopsies.

i. What techniques and instruments can be utilized to obtain tissue samples? Which instrument is pictured (**119**)?

ii. Which portion of the renal parenchyma should be sampled?

iii. What are the risks of renal biopsies, and how can these risks be minimized?

iv. When evaluating biopsy samples, several techniques may be utilized including histopathology, electron microscopy (EM), and immunofluorescent microscopy (IFM). How should samples be handled to ensure that all appropriate testing can be completed?

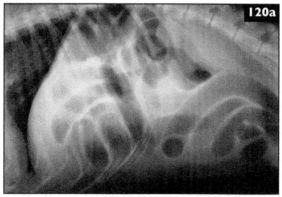

120 A 5-year-old German Shepherd dog presents with acute onset abdominal pain and lethargy. A lateral abdominal radiograph is shown (**120a**).

i. What is your diagnosis?

ii. Do you need any other tests to confirm diagnosis?

iii. What is the prognosis? Is surgery a reasonable consideration?

119

119i. Blind percutaneous, ultrasound-guided percutaneous, laparoscopic, keyhole and open techniques can all be performed, most commonly utilizing Tru-Cut biopsy needles (**119**) or Franklin-modified Vim Silverman needles. When the open surgery technique is utilized, wedge biopsies can also be collected.
ii. Renal cortical tissue should be collected for evaluation of glomerular disease.
iii. The most common complication is hemorrhage. The needle biopsy instrument should be isolated to the cortex and either directed along the long axis or through the short axis at either the cranial or caudal pole. The needle should not cross the corticomedullary junction. Collection of medullary tissue is unnecessary. The medulla is well vascularized and damage to an arcuate artery can lead to infarction and subsequent fibrosis. Clot formation can occur within the renal pelvis and lead to hydronephrosis; therefore, postoperative fluid diuresis is recommended.
iv. Samples should be at least 10 mm in length and collected using 16- or 18-gauge biopsy needles. A minimum of two renal cortical biopsies should be collected and, to ensure that samples are adequate, at least five glomeruli should be visualized (using a dissecting microscope) per sample. One sample should be fixed in buffered 10% formalin for histopathology. Samples for EM should be placed in 3% glutaraldehyde within 5 minutes. For IFM, samples should be frozen or placed in ammonium sulfate-N-ethylmaleimide (Michel's transport media).

120i. Mesenteric volvulus.
ii. Clinical signs are non-specific and rapidly progressive. However, radiographic signs of uniform gaseous distension of the entire intestine from the cardia of the stomach to the descending colon and normal position and size of the stomach are indicative of mesenteric volvulus. Moreover, if mesenteric volvulus is suspected, surgery should not be delayed by diagnostic tests because the intestinal hypoxia, due to the occlusion of the cranial mesenteric artery, results in necrosis of the intestinal wall (**120b**). This condition is rapidly progressive and death results from hypovolemic, septic and toxic shock.
iii. Prognosis for recovery is usually grave; when the diagnosis is clear on radiographs, most of the intestinal tract is ischemic and necrotic and the patients are usually euthanized. However, the only possibility of a successful outcome is with emergency surgical intervention. Surgical options are derotation alone or

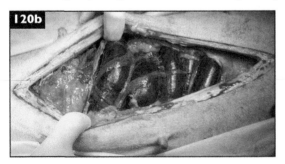

derotation plus resection and anastomosis. If only a portion of the intestine is torsed, resection and anastomosis may be performed without derotation of the torsed portion.

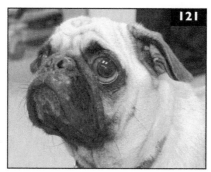

121 A 4-year-old castrated, male Pug presents for inability to eat or open the mouth (121). Pain is elicited upon palpation of the dorsal aspect of the head and with attempts to open the jaw.
i. Name the differential diagnosis.
ii. Describe how a diagnosis can be made.
iii. What are the recommended therapeutic options?

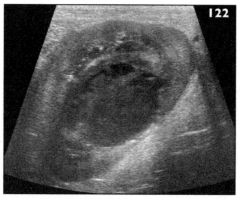

122 A 7-year-old intact, female Shih Tzu presents for evaluation of vomiting, anorexia and abdominal pain. An abdominal ultrasound is performed. An ultrasonographic image of the left kidney is shown (122). The left renal pelvis is severely dilated and filled with hyperechoic material. A large ureteral calculus is detected within the left ureter causing a chronic outflow obstruction.
i. When is nephrectomy indicated?
ii. What additional diagnostic studies should be performed prior to left sided nephrectomy?
iii. What structure should be identified and preserved while performing left sided nephrectomy in this intact female dog?

121i. Differentials included masticatory muscle myositis, disease of the temporo-mandibular joint and polymyositis. Care must be taken to differentiate from disease of the trigeminal nerve, which can result in a dropped jaw and inability to close the mouth.

ii. Diagnosis is typically made by confirming the presence of antibodies to the IIM myofibers. A muscle biopsy can be performed, showing evidence of a mixed inflammatory infiltrate. If the process is chronic, there may be evidence of necrosis on the biopsy. Advanced imaging, such as CT or MRI, can show irregular multifocal areas of enhancement in the muscles of mastication.

iii. An immunosuppressive dose of prednisone (1–2 mg/kg twice daily) is the treatment of choice. The course is prolonged, with a slow taper schedule after approximately 1 month of high-dose therapy.

122i. Nephrectomy is performed when a kidney is adversely affecting the health of an animal, usually because of severe infection, trauma or hydronephrosis. In this case, severe infection is suspected and hydronephrosis is present. The fluid within the dilated renal pelvis is hyperechoic, leading to a suspicion of pyelonephritis. Hydronephrosis and infection commonly result from renal or ureteral calculi.

ii. Prior to unilateral nephrectomy, the renal function of the remaining kidney must be determined. Evaluation of renal function can be performed with a nuclear scintigraphy glomerular filtration rate study. Urinalysis, serum biochemistry profile, and hematology profile should also be performed. In a dog with obstruction of a single ureter, azotemia is not expected in a well-hydrated, well-perfused dog. Obstruction of a single ureter does not usually cause uremia unless the contralateral kidney is not functioning normally. Urine specific gravity combined with physical examination findings may assist in diagnosing dehydration.

iii. The left ovarian vein drains into the left renal vein rather than the caudal vena cava. The ovarian vein should be identified and the renal vein should be ligated and transected distal to its origin, preserving the venous drainage of the left ovary. The arterial supply of the kidney originates from the aorta and should be isolated and ligated close to the aorta. Vessels larger than 2 mm in diameter should be double ligated. Vessels larger than 3–4 mm should be doubly ligated and transfixed. The artery and vein should be separated and ligated individually because of the possibility of ligature slippage or the formation of an arteriovenous fistula (Rawlings, 2003).

123 A chest wall excision has been performed for treatment of a vaccine-associated fibrosarcoma on the lateral thorax of a cat. Insufficient native tissues remained to assist with chest wall closure and the decision was made to use synthetic mesh. Polypropylene mesh was used in this case (**123**).

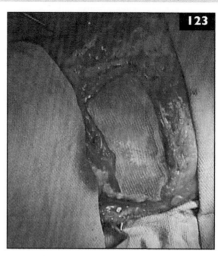

i. What properties do Prolene and Marlex mesh have that make them good/poor choices for use in thoracic wall reconstruction?
ii. What properties does polytetra-fluoroethylene (PTFE) have that make it a good/poor choice for use in thoracic wall reconstruction?

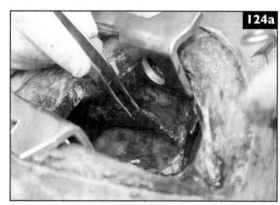

124 Surgery is underway for treatment of a thoracic foreign body and associated pyothorax in a large breed dog. A median sternotomy has been performed as an approach to the thorax in order to perform a complete exploratory and thorough thoracic lavage (**124a**).
i. What are the advantages and disadvantages of using wire or suture for sternotomy closure?
ii. What suture/wire configuration is recommended for the closure of median sternotomy?

Answers: 123, 124

123i. Prolene mesh is a double knitted polypropylene mesh. The double knitted nature of Prolene mesh makes it resistant to stretch in all directions. Marlex mesh is also a polypropylene mesh but is not double knitted. Marlex mesh has unidirectional resistance to stretch. Both Prolene and Marlex mesh have a major pore diameter between 0.6 and 0.9 mm. This pore size allows granulation tissue to grow into the pores and the mesh becomes incorporated into the tissues as the animal heals. Because of the pore size found in Prolene and Marlex meshes, they are not impermeable to fluid or air. Therefore, if tissues break down over the mesh, a pneumothorax could result. To improve the seal, omental pedicle flaps can be placed on the pleural surface of the mesh (Liptak, 2008). Infection associated with mesh application has been reported and may require removal of these non-absorbable implants.

ii. PTFE is not a woven or knitted material. It has a very small pore size (20–25 μm) and is therefore impermeable to fluid and air. Pneumothorax may be prevented with the implantation of this material. Because of the small pore size associated with PTFE, granulation tissue is unable to grow into the implant. Instead, the PTFE is encapsulated rather than incorporated. PTFE is very expensive and is not often used in large quantities in veterinary medicine.

124i. Debate exists regarding the superiority of one closure material over another. Both suture and stainless steel orthopedic wire are appro-priate closure materials for median sternotomy. Bio-mechanically, no difference was detected in displacement or in distractive forces in median sternotomies closed by the two different materials when tested up to 400N. When loaded to failure, stainless steel orthopedic wire tolerates a greater force than suture (Gines, 2011).

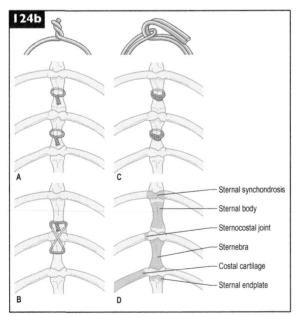

ii. A figure-of-eight pattern using twisted orthopedic wire surrounding the sternal synchondrosis is the most stable suture/wire pattern (**124b** – B). Double loop cerclage centered on the middle of the sternebrae should be avoided as this pattern has been shown to be prone to wire failure at high loads (**124b** – D).

Sternal synchondrosis
Sternal body
Sternocostal joint
Sternebra
Costal cartilage
Sternal endplate

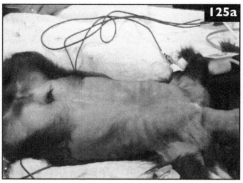

125 For the animal in **125a**:
i. What treatment options exist for this disorder?
ii. Name a severe immediate complication of treatment.

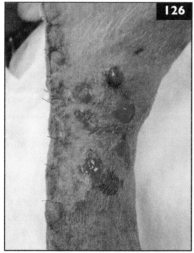

126 The hindlimb of a dog is pictured (**126**) approximately 1 week following a mass removal with primary closure.
i. What procedure was performed in addition to the mass removal?
ii. Why was this procedure performed?
iii. What is the recommended orientation and spacing?

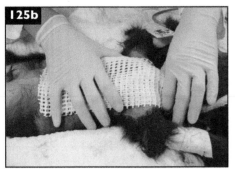

125i. Treatment of pectus excavatum is either non-surgical or surgical depending on the severity of clinical signs. If the deformity is mild and does not cause clinical signs, no treatment is indicated. If the animal is clinically affected and surgery is indicated, external or internal splinting is performed. External splint placement is the most frequently performed treatment option and is appropriate in young dogs and cats (125b). Sutures are preplaced around the sternum and fed through a custom made ventrally located splint, applying traction to the sternebrae. The patient is re-checked weekly (and radiographed) to assess progression of the correction, as well as the splint fit and skin and suture site care underneath the splint. A third option, described in a mature cat, is to reduce the deformity surgically and use an internal splint (Risselada, 2006).

ii. In animals with pectus excavatum, the lung parenchyma has chronically been collapsed. In these animals care must be taken during pulmonary inflation because re-expansion pulmonary edema after acute reduction of the deformity may occur. Another immediate complication would be damage to intrathoracic structures (lung, heart, internal thoracic arteries, lungs) while passing the suture around the sternum.

126i. Multiple releasing incisions were performed.

ii. This procedure was performed for tension relief. Mass removals on extremities often lead to excessive tension, as the skin on the extremities is less mobile than that on the trunk. Multiple releasing incisions may work well as tension relief to allow wound closure. However, circulatory compromise to the incised skin is possible by transecting cutaneous vessels. Care must be taken when performing this technique.

iii. Multiple releasing incisions should be made parallel to the long axis of the wound. The releasing incisions should be no closer than 1 cm from the wound, and should be no more than 1 cm in length. Multiple rows of releasing incisions can be made approximately 1–2 cm from the preceding row and placed in a staggered fashion. In surgery, the surgeon should periodically check tension on the wound. Once tension is relieved, no more releasing incisions must be created. The primary wound is then sutured closed and the releasing incisions remain open. The limb is covered with a non-adherent dressing and bandaged to prevent excessive motion and to protect the open wounds. The small wounds will granulate and epithelialize – healing by second intention. When using multiple releasing incisions, the result is cosmetic and successful if the original defect comprises 25% of the limb circumference or less. Results can be successful if the wound comprises 33% of the limb circumference, but the cosmetic result is less appealing.

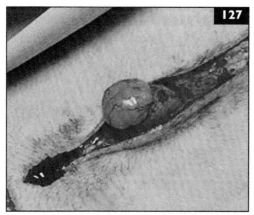

127 An incision through the skin has been created in a 7-month-old female dog undergoing ovariohysterectomy (**127**). A firm, round swelling that has grown in size over the last few weeks has been noted by the owner at the level of the umbilicus.

i. What is the diagnosis?

ii. What are the three components of this condition?

iii. What other conditions can coexist?

iv. What are incarceration and strangulation?

v. What is an omphalocele and a gastroschisis?

128 A 7-year-old spayed, female Daschund with uncontrolled protein losing enteropathy presents for acute hindlimb paresis. Advanced imaging under general anesthesia is selected to investigate the cause of paresis. Preanesthetic bloodwork reveals an albumin of 1.1 g/dL, globulin of 1.7 g/dL, and cholesterol of 80 mg/dL. Moderate ascites is suspected on physical examination.

i. What are options for providing oncotic support to this patient? List products in order of the lowest colloid osmotic pressure (COP) to the highest.

ii. What specific potential complication can occur with administration of high doses of hydroxyethyl starch solutions? Which hydroxyethyl solution is considered to be safer to administer at high doses and why?

127i. This dog has an umbilical hernia. During embryonic development the abdominal wall is formed by coalescence of the lateral, caudal and cephalic folds, with the umbilical ring remaining as a passageway for the umbilical cord. Congenital umbilical hernias are a result of a failure of fusion of the lateral folds. The majority of umbilical hernias are inherited and affected dogs should not be part of a breeding program. Airedale Terriers, Weimaraners, Basenjis, Pekingese, and Pointers are at a greater risk of umbilical hernia.

ii. There are three parts to a hernia: the ring, the sac and the contents. 'True' abdominal hernias have a peritoneal sac surrounding the hernial contents. 'False' hernias do not have a peritoneal lining.

iii. Cryptorchidism is commonly found along with umbilical hernia in male dogs. Other possible coexisting defects include cranioventral abdominal hernias, incomplete fusion of the caudal sternum and diaphragmatic hernia of various types.

iv. Incarceration occurs as a result of luminal obstruction of organs (e.g. intestine, uterus, bladder) within the hernia. Emergency surgical intervention is required in cases of acute incarceration. Strangulation within a hernia suggests that hernia contents are incarcerated and are losing viability as a result of vascular compromise.

v. An omphalocele is a large, congenital defect on the ventral midline at the level of the umbilicus that allows abdominal organs to escape from the peritoneum. Gastroschisis is a condition where abdominal organs herniate through the base of the umbilical cord and into the amniotic fluid, looking similar to an omphalocele except gastroschisis is always paramedian in location and without a peritoneal lining.

128i.

Colloidal solution	COP (mmHg)
Plasma	Low 20s
Hydroxyethyl starch 6% (in 0.9% saline)	Low 30s
Hemoglobin-based oxygen-carrying solution (Oxyglobin)	35–40
Tetrastarch in 0.9% saline	High 30s
Dextran 70*	60
25% human albumin	100–200
* Dextran 70 is no longer available in the USA due to potential for renal damage in humans.	

ii. High-dose administration of hydroxyethyl starch (>20 mL/kg/day) can be associated with development of bleeding disorders. This is thought to be associated with a dilutional coagulopathy, increased microvascular perfusion and/or decreased platelet aggregation. Tetrastarch has a lower molecular weight (MW), lower molar substitution (MS), and a higher C2:C6 ratio. The lower MW and MS limit its effect on coagulation. The higher C2:C6 ratio does not have an impact on coagulation but results in slower degradation and prolonged effect of this product.

129 A 5-year-old intact, male German Shepherd dog presents with a 2-day history of acute onset lethargy, tachypnea and abdominal distension. A right lateral radiographic projection of the abdomen was obtained (**129a**).

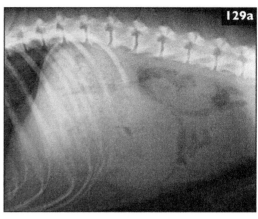

i. List the radiographic abnormalities and diagnosis.
ii. What findings on alternative diagnostic modalities can be used to confirm the diagnosis?
iii. What is the recommended treatment?
iv. What procedure may be performed concurrently?

130 A 4-year-old mixed breed dog presents for lethargy. On examination, pain was elicited on palpation of the dorsal aspect of the left scapula. The area was shaved and a small, red wound was noticed. The dog was treated with antibiotics and discharged to the owners. The following day, the dog re-presented (**130**).

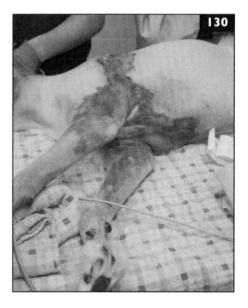

i. What is your primary differential diagnosis?
ii. What are the most likely bacteria to cause this condition?
iii. What treatment should be recommended?

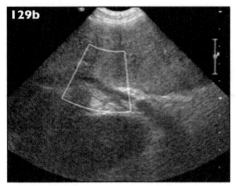

129i. A normal splenic silhouette is not present. A C-shaped mid-abdominal mass is identified. These findings are consistent with acute splenic torsion.

ii. On ultrasonographic exam, the splenic parenchyma typically has a coarse or 'lacy' appearance (129b). Thrombi may be identified in the splenic vein using B-mode, with absent flow velocity in the splenic veins on color Doppler. The identification of a triangular hyperechoic area at the hilus between the splenic veins and parenchyma has been significantly associated with the presence of an acute splenic torsion (Mai, 2006). Failure of contrast enhancement of an enlarged spleen with a corkscrew-like soft tissue mass effect (rotated pedicle) has been reported on CT (Patsikas, 2001).

iii. Splenectomy without derotation of the pedicle should be performed to prevent the release of thrombi, endotoxins and free radicals.

iv. Concurrent gastropexy may be performed to reduce the risk of subsequent gastric dilatation volvulus (Millis, 1995).

130i. The primary differential diagnosis is necrotizing fasciitis. This bacterial infection is rapidly progressive and induces significant pain with small lesions, as in this case. Necrotizing fasciitis may occur following minimal trauma to the skin or blunt trauma. It should be suspected in animals presenting with erythema, edema and severe pain. Shock and fever are often present.

ii. Streptococci Group G are the most likely bacteria to cause necrotizing fasciitis. In humans, group A streptococcus is the most likely causative agent.

iii. Immediate surgical debridement is necessary and recommended. The hallmark surgical finding is ease of separation of fascia from other tissues by blunt dissection. Tissue destruction spreads horizontally within the subcutaneous tissues. Therefore, tissue biopsy and culture should be obtained from the junction of the diseased and normal skin (not from the middle of the lesion). Cultures from the middle of the lesion may be of no use as the bacteria are advancing rapidly. The overlying skin necroses as a result of toxin-induced vasoconstriction or thrombosis. Toxic shock syndrome is commonly experienced in animals with necrotizing fasciitis and the animal should be treated aggressively. Multiple episodes of surgical debridement may be required to treat this condition adequately. Reconstructive surgery can be considered following cessation of tissue necrosis and formation of healthy tissue.

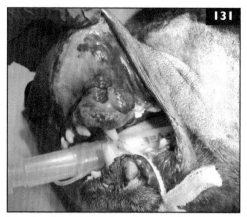

131 The oral cavity of a dog presenting for oral bleeding and halitosis is shown (131).
i. What are the most common oral tumors found in dogs?
ii. Which of these tumors carries the best prognosis and which carries the worst prognosis?
iii. What preoperative staging is recommended in this dog?

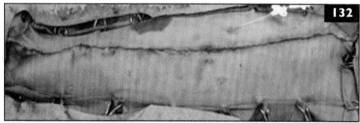

132 A surgical procedure on the ventral abdomen has been completed in an 11-year-old spayed, female domestic long hair cat (132).
i. What procedure has been performed?
ii. What is the most likely indication for this procedure?
iii. Is any further treatment required?
iv. What is the prognosis for this cat?

131i. Malignant melanoma, squamous cell carcinoma, fibrosarcoma, osteosarcoma and acanthomatous ameloblastoma are the most common oral tumors in dogs in descending order of frequency.

ii. Each of these tumors can be locally invasive (including invasion of bone). The metastatic potential varies widely among these five tumor types, with malignant melanoma and osteosarcoma being the most frequent to metastasize. Oral osteosarcomas often metastasize to the lungs, but the survival time after surgical excision is greater than that for appendicular osteosarcoma. Fibrosarcoma and squamous cell carcinoma have lower metastatic potential. Overall, squamous cell carcinoma and acanthomatous ameloblastoma have the best survival times following complete surgical excision. Malignant melanoma has a high metastatic potential but survival times often approach 1 year.

iii. Thoracic radiographs should be obtained. Oral radiographs may aid in determining the extent of the tumor. CT and MRI are superior to radiographs for assessing bony and soft tissue margins. Biopsies may be performed and should be a deep wedge of tissue by an oral approach. The biopsy should be made at a site that can be completely excised at a subsequent surgery. Lymph node palpation (mandibular) and fine needle aspirates should be performed. The medial retropharyngeal and parotid lymph nodes also drain the oral cavity and may be evaluated and aspirated with ultrasonographic assistance. The presence of normal sized lymph nodes does not exclude the possibility of metastatic disease. In approximately 40% of dogs with oral melanoma and normal sized lymph nodes, metastatic disease was detected on cytologic or histologic evaluation (Williams, 2003a).

132i. Unilateral chain mastectomy.

ii. Mammary gland neoplasia.

iii. Contralateral chain mastectomy is recommended. Some surgeons perform one-stage, bilateral chain mastectomy in dogs but this is not frequently performed in cats. Many cats do not have abundant skin to allow a bilateral chain mastectomy and closure.

iv. In cats ~85% of mammary gland neoplasia is malignant, with size of tumor, extent of surgery and histologic grade having prognostic significance. Cats with tumors larger than 3 cm in diameter had a median survival time (MST) of 4–12 months, for tumors 2–3 cm, MST ranged from 15 to 24 months and for tumors <2 cm, MST was >3 years following surgical intervention. Because of the aggressive nature of feline mammary neoplasia, it is assumed that all mammary tissue has undergone malignant transformation and should be removed (staged, bilateral chain mastectomy or one-stage bilateral chain mastectomy).

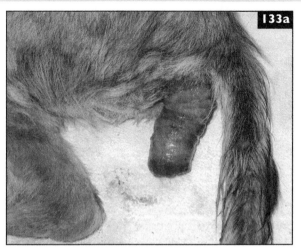

133 A 1-year-old mixed breed dog presents with rectal prolapse (**133a**).
i. How is rectal prolapse differentiated from prolapsed intussusception?
ii. How would you treat a recurrent or non-reducible rectal prolapse?

134 A 10-year-old Yorkshire Terrier presents for kidney stones. Removal of the stones by nephrotomy is planned.
i. Give two reasons why nephrotomy would be recommended.
ii. What surgical techniques are used for nephrotomy?
iii. Which nephrotomy technique is reported to disturb the glomerular filtration rate (GFR) the least?

Answers: 133, 134

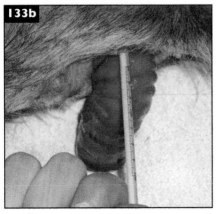

133i. Differentiation of rectal prolapse from prolapsed intussusception may be achieved by inserting a lubricated probe or gloved finger between the prolapsed rectum and the anus (133b). In the case of intussusception, cranial advancement of the probe more than a few centimeters can be easily performed between the prolapsed rectum and the rectal wall. If a rectal prolapse is present, advancement of the probe is impossible as the prolapsed tissue unites with the anal mucocutaneous junction.

ii. In these cases, colopexy is required as a definitive treatment. Colopexy is performed through a ventral midline celiotomy. Cranial traction is placed on the descending colon while a non-sterile finger inserted in the rectum ensures reduction of the prolapse. Colopexy of the descending colon is performed in the left abdominal wall 2.5 cm lateral to the midline. An incisional or a suture colopexy may be used. For an incisional colopexy, two incisions are made: the first incision is made in the antimesenteric seromuscular wall of the colon and the second in the adjacent transversus abdominis muscle. Each edge of the colonic incision is sutured to the respective abdominal incision using a non-absorbable monofilament suture material. Suture colopexy technique requires placement of two rows of six simple interrupted non-absorbable monofilament sutures between the animesenteric submucosal colonic surface and the abdominal wall. No difference exists in terms of long-term outcome between the two techniques.

134i. Nephrotomy may be indicated to remove nephroliths when infection is present or when the stones are causing an obstruction to urine flow. In some dogs, nephroliths may not cause sufficient damage to the animal's kidney to warrant a recommendation of surgical removal.

ii. The standard surgical technique in dogs has been bisection nephrotomy. In the bisection nephrotomy, the kidney is divided into halves using a midline incision through the convex surface of the kidney. A second nephrotomy technique is an intersegmental incision, designed to follow the intersegmental plane. The intersegmental plane is between the terminal branches of the dorsal and ventral branches of the renal artery of the kidney. By incising the kidney on the intersegmental plane, the interlobar arteries should be spared.

iii. Neither the bisection nephrotomy nor the intersegmental nephrotomy was found to decrease GFR in dogs (Stone, 2002). The intersegmental nephrotomy took a significantly longer amount of time to perform. Therefore, the bisection nephrotomy is recommended in dogs.

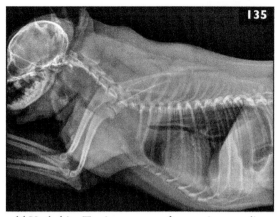

135 An 11-year-old Yorkshire Terrier presents for respiratory distress. The episode of respiratory distress was induced by an episode of extreme excitement.
i. What is your diagnosis (135)?
ii. What diagnostic tests could be advised?
iii. What treatments are available?

136 An 8-year-old spayed, female domestic short hair cat presents for evaluation of non-healing wounds on the ventral abdomen (136). The cat is noted to be indoor/outdoor and otherwise healthy according to her owners. Initially, the owners described a single exudative wound on the abdomen that had failed to respond to oral antibiotic administration after 1 month. The lesions have progressed to what you note on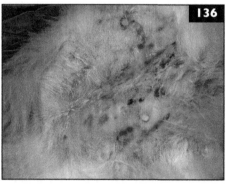
physical examination. On palpation, the wounds are highly exudative, restricted to the abdominal fat pat (which is fairly prominent in this patient) and appear to follow a cord-like distribution extending dorsally. Cytology of the exudate reveals severe pyogranulomatous inflammation. The pathologist notes several Gram-positive, acid-fast bacilli on the submitted sample.
i. Based on the information provided, what is the most likely diagnosis for this patient?
ii. What types of organisms are typically implicated in this type of infection?
iii. What treatment recommendations should be considered for this cat?

135i. The dog has tracheal collapse. The trachea is severely narrowed at the thoracic inlet.

ii. In addition to the thoracic radiographs, fluoroscopy can provide important information. Tracheal collapse is a dynamic process. Fluoroscopy provides visualization of the airway during inspiration, expiration and while eliciting a cough. Tracheobronchoscopy is another imaging procedure that allows the clinician to visualize the trachea and mainstem bronchi as the dog breathes. Tracheobronchoscopy allows the severity of tracheal collapse to be graded I–IV. Grade I indicates 25% of the tracheal lumen is collapsed, grade II indicates 50% collapse, grade III indicates 75% collapse and grade IV is completely collapsed with the dorsal and ventral tracheal walls in contact with each other.

iii. Many different treatments are available. The mainstay of medical management is antitussive medication. Sedatives to prevent excitement or anxiety may also be administered. Environmental control is quite important to prevent exposure to respiratory irritants such as smoke, perfumes, cleaning agents and dust or mold. Occasionally, antibiotics, a short course of an anti-inflammatory dose of steroid and/or bronchodilators can be used. Medical management should be exhausted before surgical intervention is provided. Surgical management of tracheal collapse includes extraluminal prosthetics such as extraluminal rings and intraluminal tracheal stents.

136i. Mycobacterial infection.

ii. Rapidly growing mycobacterial species are most commonly implicated in this type of infection in cats. Species include: *Mycobacterium fortuitum* group, *Mycobacterium chelonae/abscessus* group, *Mycobacterium smegmatis* group, *Mycobacterium phlei*, *Mycobacterium thermoresistible*, *Mycobacterium xenopi*, *Mycobacterium szulgai* and *Mycobacterium kansaii*.

iii. Radical surgical resection or extensive debridement of infected tissue is preferred; however, this may not be sufficient alone. The organisms tend to migrate along fascial planes; surgery may allow for infection to spread. Long-term antibiotic administration (doxycycline or minocycline, fluoroquinolone antibiotics) is generally recommended following surgery. Antibiotic therapy alone may lead to clinical remission; however, administration is often necessary for 6–7 months or longer. Although recurrence is common with either treatment option, long-term clinical remission may be possible with continued antibiotic administration.

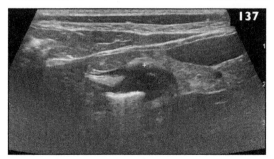

137 A 10-year-old spayed, female mixed breed dog presents for a several month history of intermittent vomiting. An abdominal ultrasound was performed (**137**) that showed a focal loss of gastric wall layers and a mass in the pylorus. An enlarged gastric lymph node was also present.
i. What diagnostics could be performed to further diagnose this lesion?
ii. What are differential diagnoses for the mass?
iii. Given that the mass is in the pylorus, what surgical options are available?

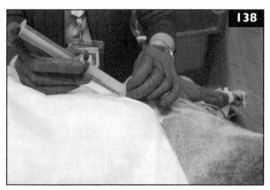

138 A male dog is being prepared for surgery (**138**).
i. What step of the preparation is being performed?
ii. What substance is being used for preparation?

137i. In order to diagnose the lesion, ultrasound guided fine needle aspirate could be attempted. Endoscopy of the upper gastrointestinal tract with biopsies is also indicated.

ii. In dogs, most gastric neoplasias are malignant and epithelial in origin. The most common gastric tumors found in dogs are adenocarcinoma, carcinoma, leiomyosarcoma, gastrointestinal stromal tumor and lymphoma. Other non-malignant differential diagnoses would include pythiosis, leiomyoma and adenomatous polyps. In cats, the most common gastric tumor is lymphoma.

iii. Depending on the biopsy results, and invasion of the mass, a submucosal resection including a 1 cm perimeter of normal tissue may be appropriate. In benign lesions confined to the submucosa/mucosa, the submucosal resection may be curative. If the mass is extensive, malignant or invading the seromuscular layer, a more aggressive resection is required. A partial resection of the pylorus can be performed for small lesions that do not involve the entire circumference of the pylorus. If the circumference of the pylorus is involved, a gastroduodenostomy (Billroth I) or gastrojejunostomy and biliary re-routing (Billroth II) procedure should be considered. The surgery (Billroth I or Billroth II) is determined by the extent of disease in the proximal duodenum. To perform a Billroth I, the entire lesion should be removed with 1–2 cm margins and preserving at least 1 cm of duodenum oral to the major duodenal papilla. If this is not possible, a Billroth II is performed.

138i. This is a male dog that is undergoing surgical preparation for an abdominal surgery. All dogs undergoing a full abdominal approach should have a routine clip and scrub of the ventral abdominal skin. In male dogs, the preputial cavity should undergo an antiseptic flush in order to decrease the bacterial load within the prepuce. In a routine abdominal exploratory in which access will not be required to the urogenital tract, the prepuce is excluded from the surgical field in order to decrease potential contamination of the surgical site. Bacteria commonly isolated from the prepuce of dogs include *Pasteurella multocida*, β-hemolytic streptococci, *Escherichia coli*, *Staphylococcus aureus* and coagulase-positive staphylococci.

ii. A two-minute flush with chlorhexidine diacetate solution (0.05% solution) is recommended for preputial cavity flush. Chlorhexidine diacetate solution has been shown to decrease the number of positive postflush cultures when compared to povidone-iodine solution (1%). Further, chlorhexidine diacetate solution does not cause increased mucous membrane irritation when compared to povidone-iodine solution (Neihaus, 2011). Detergent containing cleansing solutions, such as chorhexidine gluconate or povidone-iodine scrub, are not recommended for use on mucous membranes as they are likely to cause mucous membrane irritation.

139 i. What is this instrument (**139**)?

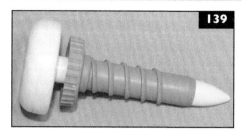

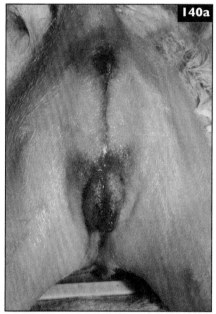

140 A 5-month-old female toy Poodle presents with tenesmus and vulvar fecal soiling since birth.

i. What is your complete anatomic diagnosis (**140a**)?

ii. What further diagnostic tests could you do to classify this type of congenital anomaly?

iii. What type of surgical procedure or procedures would be indicated to correct this congenital anomaly?

iv. What is the long-term prognosis with this condition?

139i. This instrument is a thoracoscopy cannula. This example is a disposable type. When performing thoracoscopy, one way valves are unnecessary because the thoracic wall is rigid; therefore, no isufflation is needed. Because insufflation is not necessary, airtight seals between the cannulae and body wall are not required, nor are valves to prevent leakage at the junction between the telescope and the cannula. Thoracoscopy cannulae are shorter than laparoscopic cannulae. Laparoscopic cannulae can be used for thoracoscopy if the valves are removed.

140i. Atresia ani with rectal vaginal fistula.
ii. A retrograde contrast vaginogram is indicated to document communication between the vagina and rectum (**140b**). Type I anomalies involve anal stenosis without imperforate anus. Type II anomalies consist of an imperforate anus with an anal dimple and terminal rectum lying directly beneath the anal skin. Type III anomalies involve an imperforate anus with the terminal rectum ending in a blind pouch greater than 1 cm from the anal skin. Type IV anomalies do not have an imperforate anus and have normal anal anatomy but have a blind-ended terminal rectum within the pelvic canal.
iii. The anomaly can be corrected using *in situ* anoplasty with ligation and transection or resection and over-sewing of the rectal vaginal fistula. Alternatively, the rectal vaginal fistula itself can be used to create the new anal orifice. Since concurrent megacolon and obstipation are often present, some surgeons perform a laparotomy and fecal evacuation via colotomy at the time of anoplasty.
iv. The patient is treated with stool softeners since tenesmus and rectal stricture are common following surgery. Most animals with type I or type II anomalies do not have long-term fecal incontinence following surgery. Fecal incontinence is more common in animals with type III anomalies because hypoplasia of the external anal sphincter with agenesis of the anal sacs occurs.

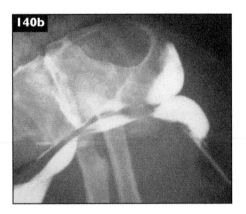

140

141 A 3-year-old intact, male English Bulldog presents for a 2-month history of difficulty urinating. The dog has a history of stone formation and had a cystotomy performed approximately 1 year ago. Abdominal radiographs are performed and multiple, faint, soft tissue to mineral opacity cystic and urethral calculi are seen. The dog is placed under general anesthesia and retropulsion of the urethral calculi is attempted (**141**).

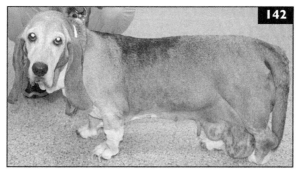

i. What study has been performed?
ii. Have all of the stones been retropulsed into the urinary bladder?
iii. What procedure should be recommended for this dog?

142 A 9-year-old intact, female Basset Hound presents for this slow growing mass on the ventrum (**142**). The mass is pendulous but firm and irregular on palpation and is related to the mammary tissue.
i. What is your diagnosis?
ii. What additional testing should be performed?
iii. What are prognostic indicators for mammary tumors in dogs?

141i. Following the retropulsion, this retrograde positive contrast urethrogram was performed to monitor for the presence of radiolucent stones.

ii. No. Multiple calculi are still present within the penile urethra at the caudal aspect of the os penis. These stones are detected as filling defects during the positive contrast urethrogram.

iii. Initially, retropulsion of the stones into the urinary bladder followed by a cystotomy was planned. Because the stones could not be retropulsed into the urinary bladder, and because the dog is suspected to be a chronic stone former, a scrotal urethrostomy is recommended. This dog is an intact male and will require castration to perform a scrotal urethrostomy. If castration is not considered for breeding purposes, the urethrostomy incision can be located in the prescrotal location; however, the dog will not have the ability to breed naturally. The urethrostomy is performed similarly regardless of location. The retractor penis muscle is freed and retracted laterally. An incision is made on midline of the urethra. Identification of the midline of the urethra can be facilitated by the placement of a urinary catheter. A 2.5–4 cm incision is made in the urethra. Several sutures are placed between the tunic of the penis to the subcutaneous tissue surrounding the urethrotomy incision in order to maintain the penis in a superficial location. The urethral mucosa is sutured to the skin. Perfect apposition of skin to mucosa is required. Bleeding is a common complication and may persist during or following urination for 10–14 days.

142i. This dog has a mammary tumor. Differential diagnoses include mastitis, cellulitis, steatitis and other subcutaneous tumors. Approximately 50% of mammary tumors in dogs are benign. The benign tumor types include fibroadenomas, benign mixed tumors, simple adenomas and benign mesenchymal tumors. The malignant tumor types include solid carcinoma, tubular adenocarcinoma, papillary adenocarcinoma and anaplastic carcinoma. The most common malignant mammary tumors are carcinomas. Sarcomas comprise approximately 10% of malignancies.

ii. Additional testing should include thoracic radiographs. Up to 50% of dogs with malignant mammary tumors also have lung metastasis. Other testing may include biopsy with histopathologic evaluation of the tissue. Histopathologic evaluation is insensitive in differentiating benign and malignant tumors. However, fine needle aspiration (FNA) is beneficial to rule out other tumors that require different excision margins, such as mast cell tumor.

Ultrasonographic evaluation of regional lymph nodes with FNA may provide evidence for or against lymph node metastasis. A minimum database of information including CBC, serum biochemistry profile and urinalysis should also be performed.

iii. Several prognostic indicators have been identified in canine mammary gland tumors. Among these are tumor size, tumor fixation to underlying tissue, skin ulceration, tumor type, tumor grade, evidence of vascular or lymphatic invasion, lymphoid infiltration into tumor, lymph node involvement and the presence of estrogen or progesterone receptors.

143 A 7-year-old castrated, male Norfolk Terrier presents for evaluation of inappetence and lethargy of 1 month duration and vomiting of 3 days duration. CBC revealed a low platelet count of 156,000/µL. Serum biochemistry profile revealed an elevated total bilirubin of 10.9 mg/dL, elevated ALP of 3,906 IU/L and elevated ALT

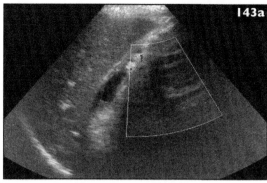

of 1,708 IU/L. The common bile duct is shown on ultrasound (**143a**).
i. Name the ultrasonographic findings and your tentative diagnosis.
ii. What surgical procedure would you advise for this patient?
iii. What are the postoperative risks/complications?
iv. What adjunctive procedure could you perform to minimize one of the risks?

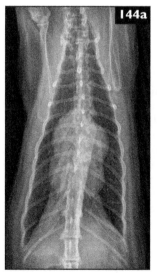

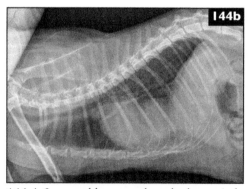

144 A 2-year old neutered, male domestic long hair cat presents for evaluation of progressive tachypnea and vomiting of 2 months duration. Muffled heart sounds were detected on cardiothoracic auscultation and orthogonal thoracic radiographs were performed (**144a, b**).
i. Describe the radiographic abnormalities.
ii. What is the purported etiopathogenesis for this condition?
iii. What concurrent diseases may be identified in dogs and cats with this condition?
iv. Describe potential treatment options and reported outcomes for this cat.

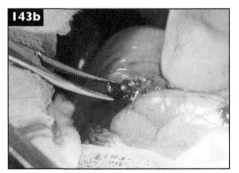

143i. The extrahepatic bile duct is markedly dilated with thickened walls. Several choleliths can be seen within the common bile duct. The gallbladder wall is hyperechoic with associated reverberation artifact and distal shadowing. The tentative diagnosis is extrahepatic biliary obstruction due to choleliths in the common bile duct.

ii. In this case, the extrahepatic biliary obstruction must be relieved. Ideally, the stones will be flushed retrograde into the gall bladder by performing an enterotomy and cannulating the major duodenal papilla. The stones will then be removed by cholecystotomy or cholecystectomy. If the stones cannot be dislodged, a choledochotomy can be performed. This procedure is performed with a longitudinal incision over the stones (**143b**). The stones are removed and the incision is closed with a small gauge suture in a simple continuous pattern.

iii. Potential complications include leakage from the choledochotomy site, compression of the common bile duct due to pancreatitis and stricture formation at the site of the choledochotomy. Of these, the most likely complication is dehiscence of the choledochotomy site because the tissue of the common bile duct is very thin and can be friable.

iv. Stenting the common bile duct may decrease the risk of short-term postoperative complications.

144i. On radiographs, the cat has an enlarged cardiac silhouette and loss of distinction between the heart and the diaphragm. These findings are consistent with a peritoneopericardial diaphragmatic hernia (PPDH).

ii. This is an uncommon congenital malformation caused by failure of formation or fusion of the septum transversum. Prevalence of PPDH is 0.025% of dogs and 0.015% of cats seen at two veterinary teaching hospitals (Burns, 2013). Proposed mechanisms include: (1) prenatal trauma to the septum transversum or the site of fusion at the pleuroperitoneal folds; (2) failure of fusion of the lateral aspects of the pleuroperitoneal folds and ventromedial aspect of the pars sternalis; or (3) aberrant development of the dorsolateral aspects of the septum transversum.

iii. Concurrent primary cardiac defects were identified in 31% dogs and 50% of cats for which echocardiography was performed (Burns, 2013).

iv. Surgical intervention by ventral midline celiotomy, with partial caudal sternotomy if necessary, reduction of herniated contents and herniorraphy has reported to resolve clinical signs in 85.3% of patients (Burns, 2013). Pericardium may be used to reconstruct the diaphragm in cases of moderate to severe diaphragmatic agenesis. A short-term postoperative mortality rate of 3.2–14% has been reported.

145 Lateral and ventrodorsal radiographs were made of a 5-year-old intact female Chihuahua (**145**). The owners complained of two large ventral swellings that had been present 2 months. The owners noticed that the swellings fluctuate in size and though they do not seem painful, the dog occasionally has difficulty urinating. Aside from the swellings on the caudal ventrolateral abdomen, the physical examination was normal.
i. What is your diagnosis?
ii. What approaches could be used for surgical repair?
iii. What are the most common complications after surgery?

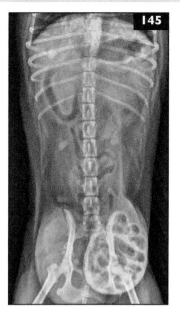

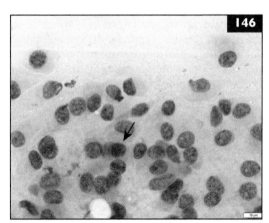

146 Aspirate from a subcutaneous mass near the elbow of a 12-year-old castrated, male Labrador Retriever is shown (**146**).
i. What is your top differential for the mass given the cytologic appearance?
ii. Identify the cell at the tip of the arrow.
iii. What characteristic of the tumor is predictive of a good prognosis independent of histologic grade (assuming surgical margins are clean)?

145i. Bilateral inguinal hernias with bladder herniation on the right and intestinal herniation on the left. Cystic calculi are present in the bladder, which is present in the right hernial sac. Inguinal hernias can be either direct or indirect. Indirect inguinal hernias occur when the hernia contents pass through the inguinal ring into the vaginal process. Direct hernias occur when the hernia contents pass through the inguinal ring but do not pass through the vaginal process and, instead, herniate next to the vaginal process. Direct hernias are uncommon. Middle-aged, intact bitches are at higher risk of inguinal hernia formation as sex hormones may weaken the inguinal ring musculature.

ii. Surgical repair could be performed by a ventral midline celiotomy or by incising over each inguinal ring. Because of the herniated bladder, need for a cystotomy, herniated intestines and bilateral nature, the best approach in this case would be a ventral midline approach. Further, if desired by the owners, a spay can be performed through this approach.

iii. Assuming no visceral strangulation, the most common complications are swelling from either seroma or hematoma formation from lack of appropriate dead space closure. Impingement of nerves (genital branch of the genitofemoral nerve) or blood vessels (genital branch of the genitofemoral artery and vein or the external pudendal artery and vein) may also occur if closure of the hernia is too tight.

146i. The cytologic appearance of this sample is classic for a perivascular wall tumor. These tumors are thought to arise from the pericytes surrounding blood vessels and were previously called hemangiopericytomas.

ii. The cell at the tip of the arrow is a crown cell, which is a cytologic feature unique to perivascular wall tumors. Typically, the cells do not display significant atypia, usually exhibiting only mild anisocytosis and anisokaryosis.

iii. Perivascular wall tumors that are <5 cm in diameter at the time of diagnosis were shown to have a good prognosis independent of histologic grade if surgical margins were clean (Stefanello, 2011). Perivascular wall tumors tend to recur locally, although distant metastasis has been rarely reported. These tumors occur more often on the extremities than the trunk and tend to be smaller in size when detected on the limbs.

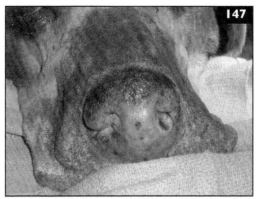

147 A 9-year-old neutered, male Labrador Retriever presents for evaluation of a mass of the nasal planum (**147**).
i. What is the most common neoplasia of the canine nasal planum?
ii. What diagnostic work-up should be recommended?

148 A 2-year-old spayed, female mixed breed dog presents for a swollen area and associated draining tract on the lateral trunk. The dog lives in Louisiana, USA and often swims in nearby ponds. The remainder of the physical examination is normal. No bloodwork abnormalities are found. You plan to perform a biopsy.
i. What pathogen do you suspect?
ii. What diagnostics will you run from your biopsy samples and what special stain will you request for histopathologic examination?
iii. What treatment will you recommend for this pathogen?

147i. The most common neoplasia of the canine nasal planum is squamous cell carcinoma. This tumor is often seen on or near the alar folds of the nares.

ii. Preoperative evaluation should include serum biochemistry profile, hematology profile, thoracic imaging (radiographs or CT) and aspiration of regional lymph nodes (submandibular). A biopsy, impression smear or aspirate of the mass itself may also be performed. Often, the extent of the tumor can be defined using CT. The CT is then used to determine the level of resection, which should include approximately 1.5 cm of normal tissue surrounding the tumor (Lascelles 2004). Consideration should be given to removal of the submandibular and medial retropharyngeal lymph nodes. If this is to be performed, the lymph nodes should be removed prior to the tumor removal so the incisions are not contaminated with neoplastic cells. The dog will need to be positioned in dorsal recumbency for lymph node removal. Following lymph node removal, the dog can be rotated into sternal recumbency for the nasal planectomy.

148i. Because of the dog's geographic location and history of swimming in ponds, *Pythium insidiosum* should be considered. *P. insidiosum* is an oomycete that infects animals mainly in temperate, tropical or subtropical climates. This oomycete requires an aqueous environment to sporulate and the resultant zoospores are attracted to hair, broken skin or open wounds. Many animals infected with *P. insidiosum* have a history of exposure to water.

ii. Several wedge biopsy specimens should be obtained from the lesion. Cultures for aerobic and anaerobic bacteria, fungi, mycobacteria and oomycetes should be performed on a portion of the tissue. Histopathologic examination should be performed on the biopsy specimen. Special staining should be performed with Gomori methenamine silver (GMS) stain. The GMS stain is particularly useful in screening for fungal organisms. Diagnostic imaging of the dog should be performed including evaluation of regional lymph nodes. Fine needle aspirates should be performed of the lymph nodes if they are enlarged. Evaluation of the aspirates should include GMS staining. Since infection with the oomycete *P. insidiosum* is suspected, ELISA-based evaluation of anti-*P. insidiosum* antibody concentrations should be performed. Advanced imaging, such as CT including IV administration of contrast, has proven helpful (Thieman, 2011) in surgical planning and may indicate extension of the disease.

iii. Surgical excision is recommended. Medical therapy may be attempted with itraconazole and terbinafine but less than 20% of animals respond to this treatment. Surgical excision with 5 cm margins and two facial planes of depth has been recommended (Thieman, 2011).

149 An 11-year-old castrated, male Standard Poodle presents for removal of a jejunal mass. Jejunal resection and anastomosis is performed with no immediate complications. To provide postoperative nutrition, a feeding tube is placed.

i. What is the most common complication encountered when providing enteral nutrition to patients in hospital?

ii. What are the indications and contraindications to placing a gastrostomy tube? What complications can occur with gastrostomy tubes?

iii. What are the indications for placing a jejunostomy tube?

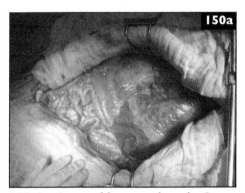
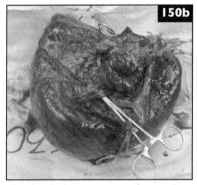

150 An 8-year-old neutered, male German Shepherd dog presents for 4 days of lethargy, discolored urine and decreased appetite. On abdominal palpation a cranial abdominal mass was found. On abdominal ultrasound, the origin of the mass was determined to be spleen. An abdominal explore was subsequently performed (**150a, b**)

i. Give your tentative diagnosis for the splenic disease.

ii. What is the explanation for the discolored urine?

iii. What diagnostics could have been added to abdominal ultrasound to evaluate the diagnosis further?

iv. What is the recommended treatment?

Answers: 149, 150

149i. Diarrhea is the most common complication associated with tube feedings and can occur due to a number of factors including: hypoalbuminemia, concurrent administration of antibiotic therapy, feeding a high-fat and/or hyperosmolar diet, feeding infected food and complications associated with underlying disease. Antibiotic administration may be the most important factor and can lead to overgrowth of enterobacteria, overgrowth of *Clostridium difficile* and decreased amounts of short-chain fatty acids. Other common complications include tube obstruction, inadvertent tube displacement/removal, aspiration, leakage through the ostomy site, and gastric pressure necrosis (with percutaneous endoscopic gastrostomy and gastrostomy tubes).

ii. Gastrostomy feeding tubes are indicated when nutritional support is required long term. This type of feeding tube should be used in patients with normal gastrointestinal motility and function. Gastrostomy tubes are contraindicated in patients with a high likelihood of ongoing and persistent vomiting, with gastrointestinal obstruction, with decreased consciousness and high risk of aspiration and those with infiltrative disease of the stomach (inflammation, neoplasia, etc.). For proper placement, the stomach needs to be apposed to the body wall. If a large amount of peritoneal effusion, mass/space-occupying lesions, adhesions or infiltrative disease interfere with close apposition of the stomach to the body wall, a different type of feeding tube should be selected.

iii. Jejunostomy tubes are indicated in patients with normal small bowel and colonic function who cannot tolerate feedings orad to the duodenum. Patients with pancreatitis, gastric outflow obstruction, gastroparesis, proximal small bowel/duodenal obstruction, partial gastrectomy/pylorectomy and those at an increased risk for aspiration are examples of ideal candidates for jejunostomy tube placement.

150i. This dog has a chronic splenic torsion. Acute splenic torsion often causes abdominal pain, collapse and shock. Chronic splenic torsion may have intermittent abdominal pain, vomiting, anorexia, abdominal distention, weight loss, polyuria and polydipsia.

ii. Hemoglobinuria is often detected in dogs with splenic torsion. Other differentials for hemoglobinuria include immune-mediated hemolytic anemia, caval syndrome and babesiosis.

iii. Doppler assessment of the pedicle of the spleen (splenic artery and vein) is performed to assess if blood flow is present and to provide the definitive diagnosis of a splenic torsion.

iv. Splenectomy is performed without derotating the spleen. The entire pedicle should be removed, including a thrombus if present.

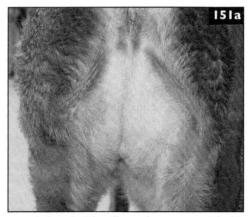

151 A 4-year-old spayed, female Bloodhound presents with this perineum (151a).
i. What is your diagnosis?
ii. What are the most common clinical signs associated with recessed vulva?
iii. What signalment is most commonly associated with recessed vulva?
iv. What surgical procedure, if indicated, can be performed for treatment?

152 A 1-year-old intact, male Golden Retriever presents for chronic weight loss, decreased appetite, vomiting and intermittent diarrhea. Clinical signs are waxing and waning but progressive in nature. On physical examination, the patient has a body condition score of 1–2/9 and a mass noted on palpation of the mid-abdomen. At the time of exploratory laparotomy, an intussusception is identified. Jejunal resection and anastomosis is performed with no immediate complications. The patient has an uneventful recovery from anesthesia.
i. Provide a postoperative nutritional plan.
ii. Which bloodwork values should be monitored postoperatively?
iii. Which potential bloodwork derangement is of particular concern in this patient? How is this complication treated?

Answers: 151, 152

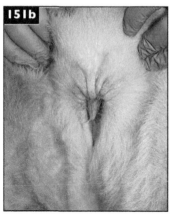

151i. This dog has a recessed vulva. Only when the skin is elevated dorsally can the vulva can be seen (**151b**).

ii. The most common clinical signs of a recessed vulva are perivulvar dermatitis, urinary incontinence and chronic urinary tract infection. Other clinical signs may include pollakiuria, irritation and vaginitis (Hammel, 2002).

iii. Most dogs that develop clinical signs associated with recessed vulva will develop those signs in the first year of life. Most dogs presenting for recessed vulva will be medium to giant breed dogs. Although previously suspected, sexual status (prior ovariohysterectomy) does not seem to influence the development of recessed vulva (Hammel, 2002).

iv. If indicated by clinical signs, the surgery of choice is a vulvoplasty (also known as episioplasty). In this procedure, a crescent-shaped portion of skin is removed from dorsal to the vulvar commissure. The skin excision continues laterally on either side and extends slightly ventrally to the thigh. The defect is closed with subcutaneous and skin sutures. This procedure results in an 82% owner satisfaction rate (Hammel, 2002).

152i. This patient is at significant risk for developing 're-feeding syndrome' due to chronic malnutrition (associated with chronic intussusception). To best avoid this complication, slow institution of alimentation is recommended. The resting energy requirement (RER) should be calculated using one of two formulas:

RER (kcal/day) = 70 × (current body weight in kg)$^{0.75}$

or RER (kcal/day) = (30 × current body weight in kg) + 70. Initial alimentation should be ~25% of total RER administered over the first 24 hours and gradually increased over the next 3–5 days until full RER is reached.

ii. Serum phosphorus, glucose, potassium and magnesium levels should be monitored at least daily for at least 5 days. PCV should be measured if hypophosphatemia is present.

iii. Hypophosphatemia is the most significant manifestation associated with 're-feeding syndrome'. Phosphate supplementation in at-risk patients is appropriate and can be achieved by supplementing enteral or parenteral formulations with phosphorus (estimated daily requirement in a dog is 75 mg/kg). In cases in which severe hypophosphatemia is present, more aggressive measures are required. Intravenous potassium phosphate or sodium phosphate at 0.01–0.06 mmol/kg/h can only be administered as an additive in IV fluids that do not contain calcium, due to the risk of forming calcium phosphate precipitate. Continuous rate infusion should be administered until phosphorus has normalized or is >2 mg/dL. Serum phosphorus and calcium levels should be monitored at least every 6–12 hours. Severe hypophosphatemia can result in intravascular hemolysis and lead to anemia, which may require administration of packed red blood cells or whole blood.

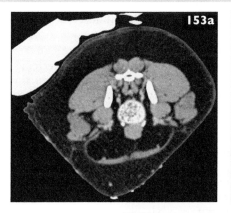
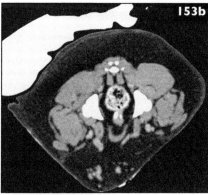
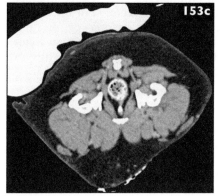

153 A 9-month-old female mixed breed dog presents for urinary incontinence.
i. What radiographic study is shown (153a–c)?
ii. Describe the radiographic abnormalities in the study shown.
iii. How is this condition best diagnosed?
iv. List the surgical procedures reported to address this condition.

154 A 9-year-old intact, male Doberman Pinscher presents for evaluation of caudal abdominal distention. The owners describe occasional urine leakage and a red discoloration of the urine. On abdominal palpation a mass lesion is appreciated but no abnormalities are palpable on rectal examination. You suspect a prostatic cyst.
i. How will you confirm your diagnosis?
ii. What are the treatment options for paraprostatic cysts?

153i. The images are from a contrast enhanced CT examination (CT excretory urography).

ii. The contrast enhanced CT reveals both ureters running parallel to the urethra and terminating caudal to the trigone. This position would be considered ectopic. Neither ureter demonstrates the traditional ureteral hook terminating in the trigone of the urinary bladder. The study is diagnostic for bilateral ectopic ureters.

iii. Ectopic ureters can be diagnosed by CT excretory urogram (as described above). Additionally, excretory urography (radiographs), retrograde vaginourethrography, transurethral cystoscopic evaluation, surgical exploratory and fluoroscopic excretory urography can be used. One study compared cystoscopy and excretory urography and found that cystoscopy correctly identified all ureters while radiographs correctly identified 78.2% of the ureters (Cannizzo, 2003). Evaluation of the kidney should be performed in addition to cystoscopy by either abdominal ultrasound, glomerular filtration rate or excretory urography.

iv. Several surgical procedures are reported in the treatment of ectopic ureters, including: neoureterostomy with ligation of the distal ureteral segment; neoureterostomy with resection of the distal ureteral segment and trigonal reconstruction; extravesicular ureteral transplantation (neoureterocystostomy) with transverse pull through technique; cystoscopic-guided laser ablation of the ectopic ureter and nephroureterectomy.

154 i. Abdominal radiographs will often demonstrate a caudal abdominal or pelvic lesion of soft tissue opacity; mineralization may completely outline the cysts, even with attachment to the prostate in some animals. Ultrasound will reveal a fluid-filled mass that creates the appearance of a second bladder. Aspiration of the mass should be performed cautiously as leakage of fluid may be ongoing after sampling and can cause a chemical peritonitis. Cytology is rarely helpful outside the presence of infection.

ii. Ultrasound-guided aspiration of the cyst in combination with castration may yield resolution. Definitive treatment typically consists of complete resection of the cyst, or partial resection with omentalization of the remaining cystic material.

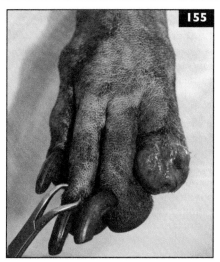

155 A photograph of the paw of a 6-year-old spayed, female Giant Schnauzer is shown (155).

i. What additional diagnostics would you perform?

ii. What surgical procedure would you recommend?

iii. What prognosis is associated with your most likely differential?

156 A 14-year-old castrated, male Rat Terrier presents with a history of anuria, enlarging abdomen and bradycardia.

i. What clinicopathologic tests are used to confirm the diagnosis of uroabdomen?

ii. What biochemistry abnormalities are common in animals with uroabdomen?

155i. Malignant melanoma of the digit is suspected. Radiographs of the paw should be performed. Approximately 80% of dogs with bony lysis have a malignant neoplasm as the cause of the mass and lysis. Squamous cell carcinoma is the neoplasm that is most likely to cause bony lysis. The radiographs of the paw will help to dictate treatment with regard to the level of digit amputation. Three view radiographs of the thorax should also be performed. Approximately one-third of dogs with digit melanomas will have radiographic evidence of pulmonary metastasis at the time of diagnosis. A fine needle aspirate (FNA) of the lymph node that drains this area should be performed. The FNA should be performed in order to detect existing metastasis. Melanomas have been known to skip lymph nodes while undergoing metastasis. Therefore, a negative FNA does not preclude the presence of metastatic disease. An abdominal ultrasound with aspiration of abnormalities detected would not be required but would be thorough.

ii. A digit amputation should be recommended. In this case, due to the size of the mass, the digit was amputated at the metacarpophalangeal joint. The extent of bony lysis present on the radiographs may help determine at which joint the digit amputation should be performed.

iii. Dogs with melanoma of the digits have a median survival time of approximately 1 year.

156i. Simultaneous evaluation of the creatinine concentration of the peritoneal fluid and the peripheral blood is used to confirm the diagnosis of uroabdomen. In uroabdomen, the creatinine concentration of the peritoneal fluid will be greater than two times that seen in the peripheral blood. BUN concentration is not useful because the urea molecule is very small and rapidly diffuses across membranes, resulting in rapid equilibration and a lack of difference in concentration between the peritoneal effusion and the peripheral blood. The peritoneal fluid in animals with a ruptured urinary tract can range from a transudate to a modified transudate, to an exudate, depending on the amount of urine in the abdomen and the amount of time that has passed from initial injury.

ii. Azotemia, hyperkalemia and hyperphosphatemia are common abnormalities seen in animals with uroabdomen. Hyperkalemia can lead to life-threatening bradycardia and should be addressed prior to anesthesia and surgery.

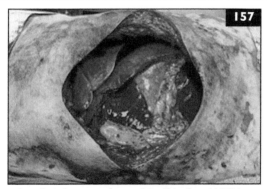

157 i. What procedure has been performed in this dog (157)?
ii. What options are reported for reconstruction of this surgical wound?
iii. What prognostic factors have been identified for pets requiring this surgery?

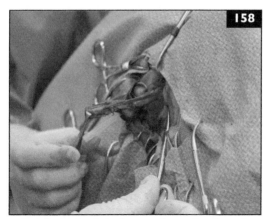

158 An intraoperative photograph is shown of a perineal urethrostomy procedure underway (158). The cat is in sternal recumbence. This procedure was performed on this cat as a result of multiple episodes of urethral obstruction.
i. What are potential complications of this procedure?
ii. How can the potential complications be avoided?
iii. What are the anatomic structures in the cat that must be transected in order to free the distal urethra sufficiently?
iv. How can the surgeon determine if the urethra has been adequately mobilized?

157i. This dog has undergone a thoracic wall resection. Typically, 3 cm or larger margins are recommended. For most thoracic wall tumors, the affected ribs are removed as well as one rib cranial and one rib caudal to the lesion. Chest wall resection involving six ribs is considered to be the upper limit for chest wall reconstruction.

ii. Muscle flaps, commercial materials or a combination of the two have been described for reconstruction following thoracic wall resection. Muscle flaps include latissimus dorsi, external abdominal oblique, transversus abdominis, pectoralis and diaphragm. The area of resection determines the appropriate muscle for reconstruction. The muscle chosen should be appropriately thick and be easily mobilized into the defect without creating excessive tension. Commercially available materials used for thoracic wall reconstruction include both synthetic and biologic materials. Synthetic materials include polypropylene mesh, polytetrafluoroethylene sheets and polyglactin mesh. The most common biologic material is porcine small intestinal submucosa.

iii. The most commonly reported neoplasias necessitating chest wall resection are osteosarcoma, chondrosarcoma and hemangiosarcoma. Dogs with chondrosarcoma have the best long-term prognosis with a survival time of over 1300 days. Dogs with osteosarcoma had a median survival time of 290 days following surgery. In dogs with osteosarcoma, increased ALP levels indicated a decreased survival time. Adjunct chemotherapy is recommended in dogs with osteosarcoma (Liptak, 2008).

158i. The most common complication in the immediate postoperative period is hemorrhage. The most common longer-term complication associated with perineal urethrostomy is stricture of the urethral stoma. Other potential complications include subcutaneous urine leakage, perineal hernia, dehiscence, urinary tract infections and urinary incontinence.

ii. Complications can be best avoided with gentle tissue handling and perfect apposition between the urethral mucosa and skin with minimal tension. Adequate dissection of the urethra is necessary to obtain tension free apposition of skin and urethral mucosa.

iii. The pelvic attachments to the penile urethra must be dissected and released to obtain adequate mobility of the distal urethra. The major attachments include the ischiocavernosus muscle and the penile ligament. Each ischiocavernosus muscle originates on the ipsilateral ischium and inserts on the penis. These muscles are best transected at their tendinous origin to prevent hemorrhage. The penile ligament is located between the ventral penis and the pubis. Minimal careful dissection is performed along the dorsal penile urethra to prevent iatrogenic damage to the innervation of the urethra.

iv. Dissection of the penis is continued cranially until the bulbourethral glands are identified. The dissection is considered complete when the bulbourethral glands are able to lie at the level of the skin without retracting into the pelvic canal.

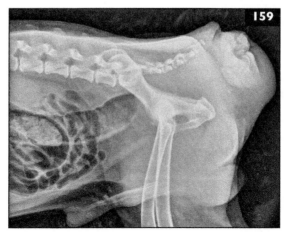

159 A 12-year-old intact, male Old English Sheepdog presents with a 2-month history of straining to defecate. When defecation occurs, the feces are ribbon-like. Additionally, the dog has not been observed to urinate for the past 12 hours and there is a progressively increasing area of swelling near the right side of the anus.
i. What is the diagnosis and the suspected pathophysiology underlying the condition (159)?
ii. Which organs may become entrapped with this condition?
iii. What techniques can be used for surgical repair?

160 A photograph of the left elbow of a 1-year-old Mastiff is shown (160).
i. What is your diagnosis?
ii. What is the recommended treatment in uncomplicated cases?
iii. What is the recommended treatment in infected cases?

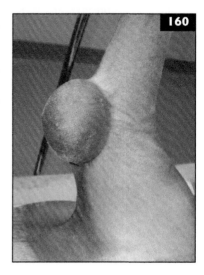

Answers: 159, 160

159i. Perineal hernia with bladder entrapment is the most likely diagnosis. This occurs due to separation or weakness of the pelvic diaphragm permitting dilation and deviation of the rectum with protrusion of various organs. The most common location for a hernia is between the levator ani, internal obturator and the external anal sphincter muscles. Hernias may occur in dogs with rectal abnormalities such as rectal deviation, dilation or diverticulum, though these conditions may be consequent to herniation rather than causal. A predisposition for herniation in non-castrated males suggests that hormones may play an important role, although this is controversial. Evidence suggests that simultaneous castration and hernia repair may help prevent recurrence. Higher numbers of relaxin receptors have been identified within the muscles of the pelvic diaphragm in dogs with perineal hernia. Relaxin from the prostatic tissue of intact male dogs may play an important role in the development of herniation. Neurogenic atrophy has been noted on EMG in some cases with localized nerve damage.
ii. Organs that may be associated with perineal hernia include the prostate, cystic paraprostatic tissue, the urinary bladder and intestinal segments.
iii. Techniques used for surgical treatment include herniorrhaphy using internal obturator muscle, superficial gluteal muscle and semitendonosus muscle transpositions, prosthetic implants and supplemental support with biomaterials (porcine small intestinal submucosa, porcine dermal collagen and fascia lata grafts).

160i. This is an elbow hygroma. Hygroma is a subcutaneous pocket of fluid that overlies the olecranon. It is likely caused by repeated application of stress on this high-pressure area while rising or lying down on hard surfaces. This condition is almost exclusively seen in large or giant breed dogs.
ii. Prevention and medical management are recommended and include soft, thick bedding and protective elbow pads. These recommendations are made when hygromas are small and non-ulcerated (uncomplicated).
iii. If the hygroma is large or becomes ulcerated and infected, more aggressive treatment is required. Infected hygromas may be managed by placing a drain into the subcutaneous pocket. This requires the limb to be prepared for surgery with a liberal clip and sterile scrub and draping. Following insertion of the drain, a padded, protective bandage should be applied and maintained to protect the exiting drain. Surgical resection is not often recommended but can be recommended for large, ulcerated, infected hygromas. If surgery is performed, sufficient skin for a tension free closure should be preserved. The skin incision and wound closure should not be located directly over the olecranon as this will increase the chance of dehiscence. Following surgery, the limb will need to remain bandaged to control dead space and facilitate healing.

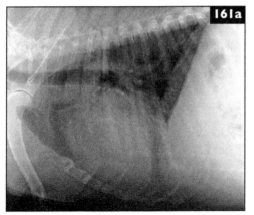

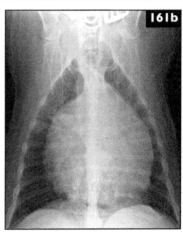

161 A 10-year-old castrated, male Airedale Terrier presents with an acute history of collapse episodes, decreased appetite and abdominal distension. Examination reveals muffled heart sounds and ascites.

i. What is your diagnosis (**161a, b**)?

ii. What is the initial treatment of choice?

iii. Name three surgical treatment options.

iv. What is the most common cause of this problem in dogs?

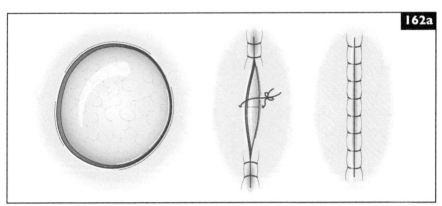

162 A circular incision was made during mass removal (**162a**).

i. What are six different techniques that can be used to close this circular defect?

ii. During the closure of the wound, a 'dog ear' was created. What are five techniques that can be used to correct the dog ear?

161i. This dog has pericardial effusion. This was diagnosed based on the globoid appearance of the heart on radiographs. Further, the physical examination finding of muffled heart sounds is consistent with pericardial effusion. The presence of ascites is likely due to right sided heart failure secondary to cardiac tamponade.

ii. A pericardiocentesis should be performed to relieve the pressure within the pericardial sac leading to cardiac tamponade.

iii. Three surgical treatments are: pericardiectomy, pericardial window, and percutaneous balloon pericardiotomy. Of these three options, percutaneous balloon pericardiotomy is the least likely to provide durable results.

iv. In dogs, pericardial effusion is most likely secondary to neoplasia (hemangiosarcoma, chemodectoma, mesothelioma and others).

162i. (1) Close in a linear fashion and excise resulting dog ears. (2) Convert circular wound to fusiform (**162b** – A). (3) Divide circular defect into three arcs and close as three separate lines (**162b** – B). (4) Combined V-plasty: in this option (**162b** – C), flaps are created on either side of a circular wound. The flaps are set at a 45 degree angle from the line of tension. The flaps are triangular (combined V-plasty), or in O-to-S-plasty the flaps are convex curves (**162b** – D). A bow tie incision is also possible. Two equilateral triangles are removed 30 degrees from the line of tension and the height of the triangles equals the radius of the circle (**162b** – E).

ii. (1) Removal of two small triangles (**162c** – A). (2) Removal of one large triangle (**162c** – B). (3) Extension of the fusiform excision (**162c** – C). (4) Removal of an arrowhead-shaped piece of skin (**162c** – D). (5) Half-Z correction (**162c** – E).

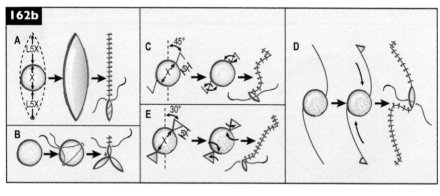

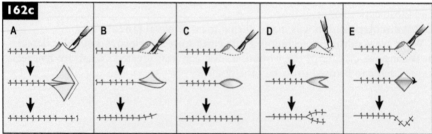

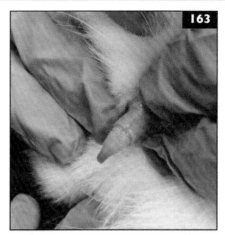

163 A male cat presents for inappropriate urination. The owners report that they adopted the cat as a young adult, approximately 1 year ago. They did not have him neutered but assumed he was neutered prior to the adoption.
i. What is a simple way to determine the neuter status of a male cat?
ii. Is this cat neutered (**163**)?
iii. Where are cryptorchid testicles usually located in the cat?

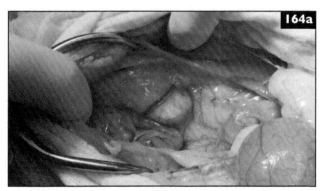

164 Obstructive ureterolithiasis is one of the most common reasons for performing ureteral surgery, especially in cats (**164a**).
i. What surgical techniques can be performed to remove ureteral stones in cats?
ii. What postoperative complications are reported with these surgical procedures?

163i. Extrusion of the penis and checking for spines on the penis is a simple way of identifying if the cat is neutered or not. Testosterone is responsible for the formation of the penile spines. The spines typically disappear within approximately 6 weeks of castration.

ii. This cat is not neutered. Spines are present on the penis.

iii. In cats, bilateral cryptorchid testicles are uncommon with approximately 75–90% of cryptorchid cats being unilateral (Steckel 2011, Yates 2003). The majority of cats have inguinally positioned cryptorchid testicles with the right and left inguinal testicles having equal incidence (Yates 2003). Abdominal cryptorchids are also reported but are rare (Yates 2003).

164i. Ureterotomy is most often performed by making a longitudinal incision over the calculus (**164b**). After stone removal the ureter is gently flushed with sterile saline to remove clots and debris and to confirm patency. The incision can be sutured longitudinally or transversely. The use of a nephrostomy tube in the postoperative period to divert urine from the surgical site has been largely abandoned because of high complication rate.

Ureteral re-implantation (neoureterocystotomy) can be performed in cases in which a ureterolith is lodged in the distal half of the ureter. The distal ureter is resected (including the stone) and re-implanted directly into the urinary bladder. After resection of the distal portion of the ureter, re-implantation can be performed using either an intravesicular technique or an extravesicular technique.

Other options for removal of ureteroliths include ureteral resection and anastomosis (performed rarely) and nephroureterectomy. Nephroureterectomy is the best option if the urinary obstruction is long standing and the kidney is no longer functioning.

ii. Development of uroabdomen and persistent ureteral obstruction are the most common postoperative complications following ureterotomy or ureteral re-implantation. Persistent ureteral obstruction is more frequently reported after ureteral re-implantation than ureterotomy, possibly because after ureteral re-implantation increased tension is present on the anastomosis. Some tension can be reduced by renal descensus, nephrocystopexy or cystopexy.

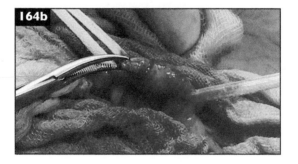

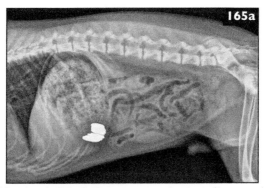

165 A 4-year-old spayed, female Pug presents for jaundice, weakness, vomiting, and discolored urine. On physical examination, generalized icterus, pale mucous membranes, pain on abdominal palpation and ptyalism are noted. Bloodwork reveals a PCV of 16% and total solids of 6.8 g/dL, a total bilirubin of 7.1 mg/dL and reticulocyte count of 345,000/µL.

i. What are the possible causes of pigmenturia in this patient? How can one differentiate between the different causes?

ii. Abdominal radiographs are performed (165a) and metallic foreign bodies (FBs) are identified in the stomach. What was most likely ingested by this patient? Why is this patient anemic?

iii. What is the treatment of choice? What should be considered prior to treating this patient for the gastric FB?

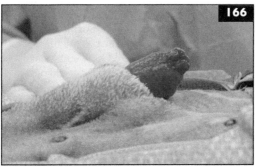

166 A 2-year-old intact, male English Bulldog presents for gross hematuria and excessive licking of the prepuce and penis.

i. What is the diagnosis (166)?

ii. What are methods of treatment for this abnormality?

165i. Pigmenturia can be caused by hematuria, hemoglobinuria, myoglobinuria and bilirubinuria. Urinalysis and plasma/serum color should be evaluated. In hematuria, plasma is clear and red blood cells (RBCs) are present in the urine. In hemoglobinuria, plasma is typically pink–red and urine is grossly red–brown and is devoid of RBCs on microscopic examination. In myoglobinuria, the plasma is clear and urine will be grossly red–brown in color and devoid of RBCs on microscopic examination. In bilirubinuria, both plasma and urine colors are orange-yellow.

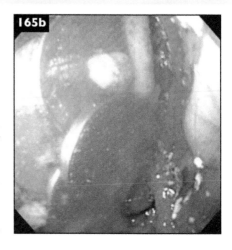

ii. A zinc coin is considered to be the most likely gastric FB. In the USA, pennies minted after 1982 have a zinc core. After the acidic environment within the stomach damages the copper coating, systemic absorption of zinc occurs. Zinc toxicosis can lead to hemolytic anemia (most often intravascular hemolysis).

iii. Removal of the FB is the treatment of choice and can be performed via endoscopy (**165b**) or gastrotomy. This patient has a severe anemia and transfusion with packed RBCs (or whole blood) should be strongly considered prior to placing the patient under general anesthesia.

166i. This dog has urethral prolapse. This condition is most common in young, male brachycephalic dogs. Diagnosis is made based on a mucosa protruding through the urethral orifice. When the mucosa is traumatized, it leads to bloody urine or blood dripping from the tip of the penis.

ii. Temporary purse string suture at the urethral orifice, urethropexy and mucosal resection have all been reported for surgical treatment. Temporary purse string and urethropexy can be performed in mild cases in which the urethra can be reduced easily by placing a urethral catheter. In urethropexy, a groove director is introduced into the urethral orifice, reducing the prolapsed urethra. With the urethra reduced, several interrupted sutures are placed through the penis into the urethral lumen, against the groove director and exiting through the penis for a total of 2–4 sutures circumferentially (Kirsch, 2002). A third method is resection of the prolapsed mucosa. This procedure should be chosen when the prolapse is long-standing or the prolapse cannot be physically reduced. Castration should be recommended as an additional surgical procedure. Urethral prolapse is suspected to be secondary to sexual excitement, masturbation and genitourinary infections.

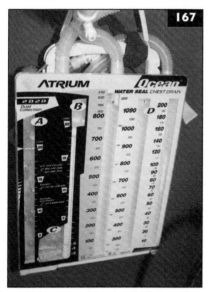

167 This portable, disposable, system is attached to a thoracostomy tube placed in a dog (167). The system is being used to evacuate the chest because of a spontaneous pneumothorax.
i. What is the function of each section of the chest drainage system?
ii. At what negative pressure should this system be set for thoracic drainage?
iii. What are the most commonly reported complications associated with thoracostomy tubes?

168 A 10-year-old spayed, female Standard Poodle is presented for lethargy, increased respiratory rate and effort, abdominal distension and non-productive retching. You suspect gastric dilatation and volvulus (GDV).
i. How will you confirm the diagnosis?
ii. Describe the surgical treatment for correction and prevention of recurrence of GDV.
iii. List three subjective and three objective methods for determining viability of the stomach wall at the time of surgery.

167i. This system has three active chambers. The far right chamber's function as a collection reservoir. The tube exiting this collection reservoir at the upper right of the photograph is connected to the patient. The second chamber is a water seal (middle). The water seal prevents air from moving into the patient. This chamber is attached to suction. The final chamber (far left) is the suction control. The amount of negative pressure applied to the thoracostomy tube is determined by the height of the column of water added to this chamber.

ii. The system is normally set at –5 to –10 cm water when attached to a thoracostomy tube. This system can be set to as much as –20 cm water.

iii. The most common complications associated with thoracostomy tubes are exudate around the stoma, premature removal, occlusion of the tube with tissue, clot or debris and subcutaneous emphysema.

168i. Diagnosis of GDV is often made based on the history, signalment and clinical signs at the time of initial presentation. Radiographs with the patient in right lateral recumbency confirm the diagnosis by demonstration of a malpositioned, air-filled pylorus (**168**). This finding has been described as a 'double bubble' or 'reverse C', which results from air accumulation in the pylorus that is separated from the air in the body of the stomach by soft tissue (compartmentalization).

ii. The aims of surgery for GDV are to re-position the stomach, resect/invaginate devitalized tissue and to create a permanent adhesion between the stomach and the body wall (gastropexy). The gastropexy should be created between the right body wall caudal to the 13th rib and the ventral aspect of the pyloric antrum. Several techniques for gastropexy have been described, including incisional, belt-loop, circumcostal, tube and incorporating.

iii. Subjective criteria for evaluation of stomach wall viability include: palpable thickness of stomach wall, color of the serosal surface, perfusion of serosal capillaries and the presence of peristaltic waves. In an experimental model, experienced surgeons are 85% accurate at assessing these subjective criteria. Objective criteria for evaluation of stomach viability include: fluorescein stain injection, scintigraphy and laser Doppler flowmetry.

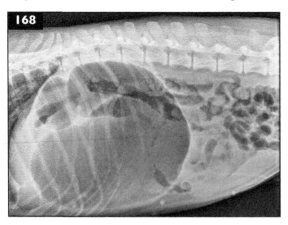

169 A 4-year-old dog presents after falling onto the ground from a deck elevated approximately 5 feet (1.5 m). On presentation, the dog is quiet and alert. You detect free fluid in the abdomen and obtain a sample. The fluid analysis is consistent with uroabdomen as the creatinine and potassium of the fluid are higher than in the blood sample.
i. What initial treatment is recommended?
ii. What imaging studies should be performed?

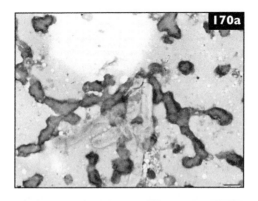

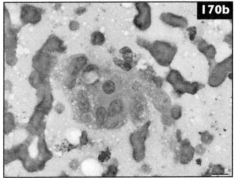

170 A scraping of a mass associated with the small intestine of a 4-year-old intact, male Labrador Retriever is shown (**170a, b**).
i. Given the cytologic appearance of the sample, what is your diagnosis?
ii. What cell is pictured in the image **170b**? How is this cell formed and what does it indicate?
iii. What is the treatment of choice for this disease? What other veterinary species may be affected?

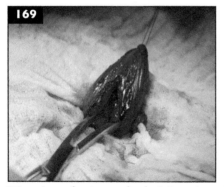

169i. Initial treatment consists of IV fluid therapy and placement of an indwelling urinary catheter while the patient is stabilized. Animals with bladder rupture often have concurrent injuries and treatment of life-threatening injuries is prioritized. The indwelling urinary catheter prevents the accumulation of urine in the abdomen. If large quantities of urine have accumulated in the peritoneum, an abdominal drain may be required. Diversion of urine and administration of IV fluids is often sufficient to improve hydration and decrease azotemia to decrease anesthetic risk. Once the patient is hydrated and stabilized, imaging studies and surgery (**169**) are planned.

ii. Plain radiographs should be performed prior to contrast radiography. Radiographs may reveal decreased serosal detail because of fluid accumulation in the abdomen and small urinary bladder. The location of urinary tract rupture must be identified using contrast radiography prior to surgery. Positive contrast cystourethrogram should reveal the presence of lower urinary tract rupture. This study will be chosen if the fluid is peritoneal rather than retroperitoneal. Small bladder ruptures may be difficult to detect and may require serial radiographs be performed. If the urethra and bladder are normal on positive contrast cystourethrogram, an IV urogram is performed to assess the ureters and kidneys. The IV urogram should only be performed in a hydrated pet.

170i. Pythiosis. The appearance of non-staining hyphae with bulbous, rounded ends and no septae is characteristic of *Pythium insidiosum*, although *Lagenidium* spp. cannot be completely excluded. Organisms may be difficult to find in cytology samples as they do not readily exfoliate, necessitating scraping of affected tissue or other aggressive means of sampling.

ii. The image shows a multinucleated giant cell which is formed by aggregation of macrophages. The presence of multinucleated giant cells indicates chronicity to the inflammation.

iii. The treatment of choice for pythiosis is surgical resection of affected tissue if possible. Response to treatment with antifungal agents has been variable with combinations of terbinafine and itraconazole or voriconazole showing more effect than single agents. Other veterinary species that have been reported include: horses, cats, cattle, sheep, birds and some captive animals (Gaastra, 2010).

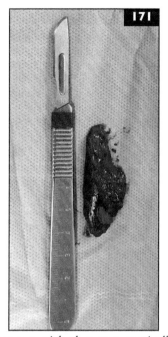

171 This photograph shows a stick that was surgically removed from a dog following esophageal perforation (**171**).
i. Describe the clinical signs consistent with esophageal foreign bodies (FBs).
ii. What is the diagnostic modality of choice to identify esophageal perforation by a FB?
iii. What are the four most common locations a FB can become trapped within the esophageal lumen?
iv. Describe the surgical approach for cervical esophageal perforation.
v. Name six potential complications following surgical treatment of esophageal perforation by a FB.

172 If an instrument has been previously sterilized by radiation, it should not be re-sterilized with ethylene oxide. Why?

Answers: 171, 172

171i. Clinical signs consistent with esophageal FB include lethargy, anorexia, hypersalivation, retching, regurgitation, restlessness and respiratory distress. One study found that the median time of clinical signs prior to presentation was 2.75 hours. Small breed dogs less than 3 years of age are over-represented. The most common objects that result in esophageal FBs are bone (30%), raw hide chews (30%), dental chew toys, fish hooks, balls and toys (Thompson, 2012).

ii. Lateral cervical and thoracic radiographs are the diagnostic modality of choice. A foreign object within the cervical or thoracic esophagus will contrast with gas opacity within the esophageal lumen and/or thorax. Evidence of cervical emphysema signifies esophageal perforation and surgical exploration is indicated.

iii. Foreign objects are most likely to become entrapped at an area of anatomic narrowing: pharynx, thoracic inlet, heart base, distal esophagus.

iv. A ventral midline cervical exploration should be performed. The incision is made from the cricoid cartilage to just cranial to the manubrium. Placement of an oroesophageal tube can aid in locating the esophagus. The area is explored, foreign material removed and the region copiously lavaged. Esophageal perforations should be repaired primarily. The margins of the wound can be minimally debrided. Recommended closure of esophageal wounds includes single or double layer, continuous and interrupted appositional patterns with monofilament suture. Placement of an active drain and gastrotomy tube is recommended.

v. Complications of esophageal FBs include: pyothorax, esophageal dehiscence following surgical repair, esophagitis, stricture, aspiration pneumonia, broncho-esophageal fistula and aortoesophageal fistula (Keir, 2010). The prognosis for survival following esophageal transthoracic retrieval of esophageal FBs was reported in one study to be 93%. The presence of mediastinitis has been associated with increased mortality (Williams, 2006).

172 Re-sterilizing an instrument with ethylene oxide that was previously sterilized by radiation may result in the formation of ethylene chlorohydrin. Ethylene chlorohydrin is highly toxic and difficult to elute.

173 A 1-year-old intact, male Chihuahua presents for evaluation of a 3 cm diameter, firm, subcutaneous mass on the caudal left ventral abdomen. It was reported that the mass was initially fluctuant and only present intermittently; however, over the previous month it had progressively increased in size and had become firm (173).

i. What is the most likely differential diagnosis for this condition?
ii. What is the typical signalment of patients with this condition and why?
iii. What is the typical presentation of patients with the acquired form of this condition?
iv. With what concurrent affliction has this condition been linked in older male dogs?

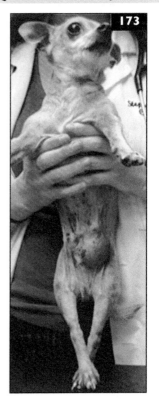

174 A 9-month-old male domestic short hair cat is presented with signs of upper respiratory noise. On oropharyngeal examination under general anesthesia the soft palate is retracted cranially and a mass located in the nasopharynx is revealed (174a).

i. What is your diagnosis?
ii. What is the etiology and pathophysiology of this disease?
iii. What are your differentials?
iv. How do you manage this case?

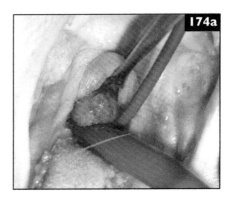

173i. This dog most likely has a congenital inguinal hernia.

ii. Male dogs more commonly develop congenital inguinal hernias, due to delayed inguinal ring narrowing secondary to late testicular descent. Several breed predispositions have been identified, although a heritable component has only been proven in Golden Retrievers, Cocker Spaniels and Dachshunds.

iii. Acquired inguinal hernias typically occur in middle-aged, intact, female dogs, with no breed predilection identified. It has been proposed that females are predisposed due to a shorter and larger diameter inguinal canal than equivalent male dogs, as well as due to estrogen production.

iv. Inguinal hernia in older male dogs has been linked with unilateral or bilateral perineal hernia.

174i. Nasopharyngeal polyp.

ii. Nasopharyngeal polyps in cats are inflammatory benign masses that originate in the middle ear or auditory tube and descend to the nasopharynx and/or external ear canal. The cause is unknown but congenital and infectious causes have been incriminated, leading to unilateral or bilateral disease. The role of inflammation and otitis media is not well understood and it is not clear if this is the result or the cause of the polyp. The polyp develops on a stalk and reaches the nasopharynx through the auditory tube; because of its size it may obstruct the upper airway resulting in inspiratory dyspnea, rhinitis and may also affect swallowing. Otitis media associated with the polyp is usually sterile. The polyp may grow through the tympanic membrane and extend to the external ear canal, leading to aural discharge.

iii. Differential diagnosis may include congenital anomalies of the nasopharynx, such as choanal atresia or stricture, nasopharyngeal foreign bodies and malignant masses, which are most commonly seen in older animals.

iv. The polyp is removed by traction of its stalk (**174b**) after cranial retraction of the soft palate or more rarely through a midline incision of the soft palate. Polyps growing into the external ear canal can be treated with a ventral bulla osteotomy and removal of the polyp at its origin.

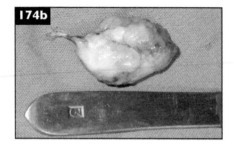

174

175 A 5-year-old spayed, female mixed breed dog presents for evaluation of urinary incontinence. The owners report that the urine dribbling started about 1 year ago and is most noticeable while the dog is sleeping.
i. What is the most likely diagnosis?
ii. What are non-surgical options for treatment?
iii. What are surgical options for treatment?

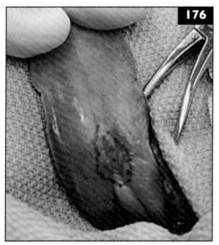

176 A 10-year-old neutered, male domestic short hair cat presents for evaluation of a mass on the ventral aspect of the tongue (**176**).
i. List differential diagnoses for this mass.
ii. List reported treatment options for the most likely differential in this case.
iii. What is the reported median survival time for cats with this condition?
iv. List the categories of glossectomy.

175i. The most likely diagnosis is urethral sphincter mechanism incompetence (USMI). USMI is diagnosed in up to 20% of spayed female dogs and is likely related to lack of hormones in the spayed female. Consideration should also be given to any process causing polyuria/polydipsia. Increase in the volume of urine produced can lead to incontinence. Additionally, urinalysis and urine culture should be performed.

ii. Non-surgical options for USMI include the administration of oral medications such as phenylpropanolamine hydrochloride, diethylstilbestrol (DES), and estriol. Estriol and DES mimic the effect of estrogens. Estrogens increase the resting muscle tone of the urethra in females. Phenylpropanolamine is an analogue of endogenous sympathomimetic amines (alpha-adrenergic agonist) and is reported to increase urethral tone in dogs. Medical therapy with alpha-adrenergic agonists and estrogen are effective in 60–90% of dogs. A different non-surgical treatment is a urethral bulking procedure. In this procedure, cystoscopy is performed and collagen is injected submucosally in the urethra leading to a smaller urethral lumen.

iii. Many surgical options are available for the treatment of USMI including culposuspension, cystourethropexy, artificial urethral sphincter, urethral intussusception and transpelvic sling.

176i. Squamous cell carcinoma is the most common tumor of the tongue in cats, frequently presenting as an ulcerated mass located on the ventral surface of the tongue and frenulum. Other less common differentials include melanoma, fibrosarcoma, eosinophilic granuloma or calcinosis circumscripta. In dogs, the most common lingual tumors include squamous cell carcinoma, malignant melanoma, mast cell tumor, hemangiosarcoma and granular cell tumor, although many tumor types have been reported to occur in the tongue (Culp, 2013).

ii. Surgical excision and/or radiation therapy have been reported.

iii. In cats with lingual squamous cell carcinoma, the prognosis is guarded to poor, with 1-year survival rates of less than 25%. The overall survival time for dogs with lingual tumors is 483 days. The median survival time for dogs with squamous cell carcinoma is 216 days and 241 days for dogs with malignant melanoma (Culp, 2013).

iv. The classification system for glossectomy includes partial or minor (excision of part or all of the body of the tongue rostral to the frenulum), subtotal (entire free portion of the tongue and a portion of the genioglossus and/or geniohyoid muscles caudal to the frenulum), near-total (resection of 75% or more of the tongue), or total (amputation of the entire tongue) (Dvorak, 2004). Subtotal, near total, and total glossectomies are considered major glossectomies.

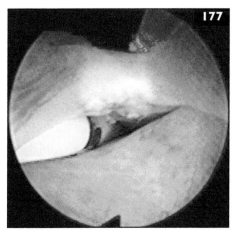

177 An 8-month-old female Golden Retriever presents for urinary incontinence. A procedure is underway for correction of a congenital abnormality (177).
i. What procedure is being performed?
ii. What prognosis is associated with this procedure?

178 An 11-year-old dog presents for testicular enlargement. One testicle is large, firm and non-painful on palpation. The remainder of the physical examination is normal.
i. What are your differential diagnoses?
ii. What additional diagnostic procedures are indicated?
iii. What is the prognosis?

179 The instruments at a practice are sterilized and stored. What is the duration of safe storage times for sterile packs stored in closed cabinets for each of the following wrappers:
i. Double wrapped muslin?
ii. Single wrapped two way crepe paper?
iii. Heat sealed paper and transparent plastic pouches?

177i. This picture is of a cystoscopic-guided transurethral laser ablation of an ectopic ureter. This procedure is appropriate for animals with intramural ectopic ureters.
ii. Approximately one-half of dogs undergoing this procedure will have urinary continence with no additional treatment. Approximately 25% of dogs undergoing this procedure will have urinary continence with an additional procedure (urethral bulking, artificial urethral sphincter). Therefore, approximately 75% of dogs undergoing this procedure will have a favorable outcome (Berent, 2012).

178i. Common testicular neoplasias include interstitial cell (Leydig) tumors, Sertoli (sustentacular) cell tumors and seminomas. Other differential diagnoses for enlarged testicle should include testicular torsion and scrotal hernia. Both of the latter two conditions should elicit pain.
ii. Dogs with a testicular tumor should undergo a CBC since some testicular tumors, mainly Sertoli cell tumors, are reported to produce estrogens that can cause myelotoxicosis. Myelotoxicosis is associated with feminization syndrome and includes anemia, leukopenia and thrombocytopenia. The prognosis with myelotoxicosis is guarded, even after castration. In addition to a CBC, three view thoracic radiographs and abdominal ultrasound should be performed. Although metastases are rare, they have been reported to occur to the medial iliac, sublumbar, inguinal, and para-aortic lymph nodes, lungs, kidneys, spleen, pancreas and liver. If abnormalities are found, fine needle aspirates should be performed.
iii. Bilateral orchiectomy is recommended because bilateral involvement is frequently reported. Both testicles should be submitted for histopathologic evaluation. Dogs with testicular neoplasia have an excellent prognosis after orchiectomy if there is no evidence of myelosuppression or metastasis. Metastases from primary testicular tumors are rare. The rate of metastasis varies by tumor type: Sertoli cell tumor 2–10%, seminoma 6–11%, and metastasis of interstitial cell tumors is very rare.

179i. Instruments in double wrapped muslin will remain sterile in a closed cabinet for 1 week. If the sterile pack is placed on an open shelf, the safe storage time is 2 days.
ii. Instruments in single wrapped two way crepe paper placed in a closed cabinet will remain sterile for 8 weeks. If placed on an open shelf, the safe storage time is 3 weeks.
iii. Instruments wrapped in heat sealed paper and transparent plastic pouches have a safe storage time of 1 year, regardless of whether it is in a closed cabinet or open shelf, provided that the wrapper is not punctured.

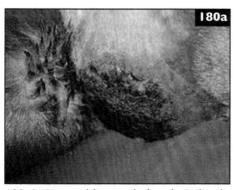
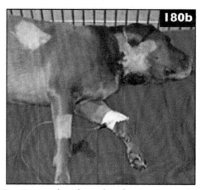

180 A 5-year-old spayed, female Labrador Retriever developed a large necrotic wound on the ventral neck 3 days after suspected crotalid (pit viper) envenomation (180a). Following debridement, a vacuum-assisted closure (VAC) device was applied over nanocrystalline silver-impregnated foam (180b).
i. What enzymes contained in crotalid venom contribute to tissue necrosis at the envenomation site?
ii. What are the antibacterial properties of nanocrystalline silver?
iii. What properties of VAC make it a desirable option in this case?

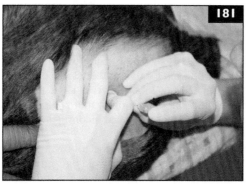

181 A 6-year-old castrated, male mixed breed dog presents for anal sacculectomy and intra-abdominal lymph node extirpation. At presentation, physical examination and bloodwork are within normal limits
i. Why would you include the regional block shown (181)?
ii. What is/are the most common drug (s) utilized for this type of block, and what consideration should be weighed to decide which drug to use?
iii. What side-effects can this block produce?

180i. Crotalid venom contains over 50 enzymatic fractions, many of which contribute to tissue damage. Proteolytic trypsin-like enzymes cause marked tissue destruction. Hyaluronidase decreases the viscosity of connective tissue, facilitating penetration of other venom components, while collagenase digests and breaks down connective tissue (Peterson, 2006).

ii. Particulate silver causes bacterial cell wall damage via alterations in DNA and RNA transcription. Nanocrystalline silver allows for sustained release of silver ions to the wound. Nanocrystalline silver-impregnated dressings have been found to be active against multidrug-resistant microbial organisms.

iii. VAC therapy has been reported to decrease interstitial edema, increase tissue blood flow, accelerate granulation tissue formation and hasten wound closure.

181i. Epidurals provide analgesia and decrease the requirements of inhalants. By administering opioids epidurally, a lower dose can be used than if the opioids were systemically injected. In addition, administration of an epidural block can decrease the requirements of analgesics postoperatively.

ii. Several drugs can be used but a typical example is preservative free morphine. The drug is delivered with a spinal needle in the lumbo-sacral space at the epidural level. Correct placement is confirmed with the hanging drop technique and lack of resistance to fluid injection. The literature suggests longer and more effective analgesia utilizing a combination of local anesthetics and opioids administered in the epidural space. Opioids exert their action by blocking Aδ and C fiber transmission, while local anesthetics act on Aδ, Aα, Aβ, B and C fibers. Local anesthetics may add the risk of interfering with motor function; therefore, it may be safer to administer opioids without a local anesthetic in surgery where motor function impairment is undesirable. At least one study reveals that using low doses of bupivacaine along with morphine will not impair motor function after splenectomy. Nevertheless, the same study was unable to report additional analgesic advantages of adding local anesthetics as opposed to administering morphine alone (Abelson, 2011). In the current case, the dog is undergoing an anal sacculectomy. With a perianal incision, a motor block is often undesirable as the motor block may lead to temporary fecal incontinence, the inability of the dog to walk and incisional contamination.

iii. Possible side-effects of opioids include the following: respiratory depression, urinary retention, pruritus, vomiting and delayed hair growth. Side-effects of local anesthetics may include motor paralysis, hypotension and weakness of respiratory muscles.

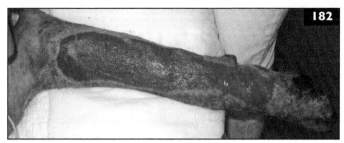

182 A 7-year-old mixed breed dog presents with severe bite wounds to the antebrachium, shown after 6 days of open wound management (**182**). You now plan to perform a free skin graft.
i. What advantages would use of a vacuum-assisted closure (VAC) bandage over the skin graft provide?
ii. Other than over skin flaps or free skin grafts, name five additional indications for VAC therapy.

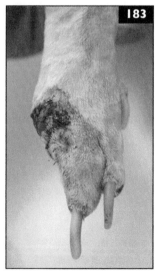

183 A photograph was taken 1 day postoperatively following the removal of an interdigital mast cell tumor (**183**).
i. What procedure has been done?
ii. Will this dog have good function of the limb?

Answers: 182, 183

182i. VAC can remove excess interstitial fluid and prevent seroma development between the graft and underlying bed. Furthermore, the VAC bandage acts as a bolster, preventing movement or shearing forces on the graft and allowing for inosculation and revascularization. VAC bandages are changed every 72 hours, thus minimizing iatrogenic disruption of the graft with bandage removal in the first 3 days after surgery. VAC provides additional benefits such as improved neovascularization and enhanced bacterial clearance.
ii. VAC therapy has been used to treat a variety of open wounds including degloving, burn, bite, puncture and as an aid in treatment of open fractures. VAC can be used to manage pin tract drainage from external skeletal fixation. VAC bandages can be placed over closed incisions following procedures at risk of interstitial edema development and incisional complications such as median sternotomy and carpal arthrodesis. Vacuum assisted peritoneal drainage has also been documented to assist in management of septic peritonitis in small animals.

183i. A phalangeal fillet (aka digital flap) was used to close the defect created during the mast cell tumor removal. During this procedure, the skin is harvested from one or more digits and used to close wounds of the distal limb. A digit adjacent to the skin defect is chosen as the donor. An incision is made along the digit and continued around the nail. The skin is elevated from the bone with care not to damage the blood supply. Sparing the soft tissues and dissecting closely to the bone protects the vasculature from being damaged. The bones of the digit are disarticulated at the metacarpophalangeal/metatarsophalangeal joint. The first through third phalangeal bones are removed. The remaining skin flap is placed into the wound bed and closed with a two layer closure. The pad may be preserved or removed. In this photograph, the pad was preserved to provide tissue to close the defect created during tumor removal.
ii. This dog should have good function of the limb. Two digits have been removed from this dog. Dogs can have a functional limb following removal of all of the digits. The older veterinary literature reports complications associated with the removal of the main weight-bearing digits (digits 3 and 4); however, recent reports state that dogs undergoing amputation of digits 3 or 4 did not have a worse outcome than dogs undergoing amputation of other digits (Kaufman, 2013).

184 A 9-year-old castrated, male Labrador Retriever presents for chronic progressive left forelimb lameness. On exam, the patient cannot fix the elbow to bear weight. No orthopedic abnormalities are detected. The dog has no response to noxious stimulus of the dorsal aspect of the paw, but response to stimulus is present when applied to the lateral aspect of digit 5. An MRI image is shown (**184**).

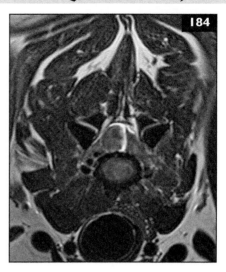

i. What is the most likely differential and what nerve is primarily affected?

ii. Name common neurologic exam findings that indicate that the central nervous system may be affected.

iii. Describe the surgical procedure required for treatment.

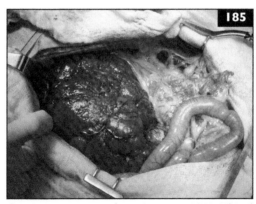

185 Surgery is underway to remove a hepatic mass (**185**). This dog will undergo a partial liver lobectomy.

i. What are surgical methods to perform a partial liver lobectomy and which will likely lead to the most blood loss?

ii. What prognostic factors have been identified in dogs with massive hepatocellular carcinomas?

Answers: 184, 185

184i. The most likely differential is a malignant nerve sheath tumor (peripheral nerve sheath tumor). Other differentials include a focal neuritis, focal lymphoma or a focal granuloma. Based on the exam findings, the radial nerve is primarily affected.

ii. If the spinal cord is involved, proprioceptive or motor deficits of the ipsilateral pelvic limb or the contralateral thoracic and pelvic limbs may be present. Horner's syndrome may be seen on the ipsilateral side due to the disruption of the sympathetic pathway. In addition, the cutaneous trunci reflex may be affected if the segments that supply the lateral thoracic nerve (C8–T1) are damaged.

iii. Amputation of the affected limb is often recommended to relieve pain associated with the tumor and prevent damage and self-trauma to the limb. Care is taken to ensure that the nerve is transected proximally to the area of the tumor. If the mass appears to be invading the spinal canal, a laminectomy or foraminotomy of the appropriate area may be required.

185i. Several different surgical techniques can be used to perform partial liver lobectomy. Techniques include stapling devices, parenchymal dissection and ligation of vessels, parenchymal dissection and hemoclip application to vessels, parenchymal dissection and occlusion of vessels with thoracoabdominal stapler, vessel sealing devices, pretied endoscopic loops, a single circumferential ligature and harmonic scalpel. In one study, the quantity of blood loss was compared following partial liver lobectomy performed with pretied suture loop, energy-based sealer-divider, harmonic scalpel, parenchymal dissection with clip application and parenchymal dissection with thoracoabdominal stapler (Risselada, 2010). This study found that all five techniques should be safe. Parenchymal dissection and clip application resulted in the highest blood loss.

ii. Dogs with massive hepatocellular carcinomas have a good prognosis following surgery. Dogs undergoing liver lobectomy have a median survival time of 1460 days while dogs not undergoing surgery have a median survival time of 270 days. The intraoperative mortality rate associated with resection is approximately 5%. Increased ALT and AST activities were associated with a poorer prognosis (Liptak, 2004).

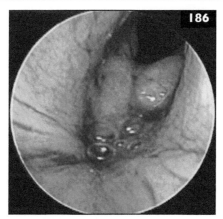

186 A 5-year-old spayed, female Cavalier King Charles Spaniel presents with a history of dsypnea, stridor and exercise intolerance and a photograph of the oropharyngeal exam is shown (186).
i. What stage of laryngeal collapse is depicted?
ii. Describe the treatment options for this stage of laryngeal collapse.
iii. Describe the surgical options for the other stages of laryngeal collapse.

187 What is the Boari bladder flap?

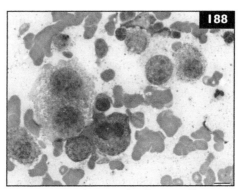

188 A cytologic examination is shown of a fine needle aspirate performed on a hairless, red, raised cutaneous lesion on the back of a 5-year-old castrated, male Boxer dog (188).
i. What is your diagnosis given the cytologic appearance of the lesion?
ii. What criteria of malignancy are exhibited by this neoplastic cell population?

Answers: 186–188

186i. Eversion of the laryngeal saccules is shown, representing stage I laryngeal collapse. Laryngeal collapse occurs secondary to chronic increased airway resistance, increased negative intraglottic luminal pressure and increased air velocity due to brachycephalic airway syndrome (stenotic nares, elongated soft palate, redundant pharyngeal tissue, pharyngeal nasoturbinates and hypoplastic trachea). Stages of laryngeal collapse range from I to III. In stage I (shown here), everted laryngeal saccules are present. In stage II laryngeal collapse, the cuneiform process of the arytenoid cartilage becomes medially displaced. In stage III laryngeal collapse, the corniculate processes collapse. The collapse of the corniculate processes leads to loss of the arch of the rima glottidis and airway obstruction.

ii. Surgical treatment includes resection of the everted laryngeal saccules as well as staphylectomy and rhinoplasty (for stenotic nares). Medical management, including weight loss and exercise restriction, can also be recommended.

iii. Patients that have a stage II or stage III collapse or that do not respond to the above treatment may require a permanent tracheostomy. A combined cricoarytenoid and thyroarytenoid caudo-lateralization has been described as successful surgical treatment for stage II and stage III collapse (White, 2012).

187 The Boari bladder flap is a full thickness urinary bladder pedicle flap used to reconstruct the distal part of the ureter. It is useful when the ureter becomes too short because of an extensive resection. The flap is harvested from a vascular portion of the dorsolateral or ventral bladder wall and is closed in a tubular shape. To determine the length of the flap required, renal descensus is performed and the distance is measured. The width of the flap should be at least 1.6 cm and should be based on bladder size. The proximal portion of the ureter should be sutured in place before the flap is closed. To reduce tension at the anastomosis, nephrocystopexy or nephropexy and psoas cystopexy are performed. Postoperatively vescicoureteral reflux is frequent; this predisposes the patient to recurrent urinary tract infection.

188i. The cytologic appearance of this sample is classic for a poorly granulated mast cell tumor. A population of round cells with numerous magenta mast cell granules is scattered among erythrocytes, non-degenerate neutrophils and plump, uniform fibroblasts, and eosinophils are observed in a clear background. Round cells have light pink to blue cytoplasm, which contains variable amounts of dark magenta granules, surrounding an eccentrically placed, irregularly round to oval nucleus.

ii. Neoplastic cells in this sample exhibit marked anisocytosis and anisokaryosis. Variable nucleus to cytoplasm ratios are also seen. Binucleation is also observed. Nuclei display a coarse chromatin pattern and contain up to seven variably sized nucleoli. Occasional angular nucleoli are observed. Histologic examination is required to determine the grade of the tumor and aspiration of regional draining lymph nodes may be helpful to evaluate the patient for spread of disease.

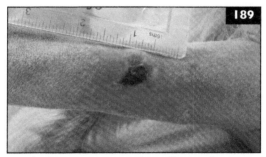

189 One of the oncologists at your practice calls you for a surgical consult on a 7-year-old castrated, male Rottweiler. You were consulted for a possible surgical resection following chemotherapy extravasation. Prior to this visit, you had performed a hind limb amputation for an osteosarcoma lesion on the proximal tibia. Adjuvant chemotherapy was initiated and the last dose administered IV, was given 7 days prior to the photograph shown (189).

i. Describe the lesion.

ii. Name the most likely drug causing this lesion.

iii. What is your surgical recommendation?

iv. Describe the recommended treatment, if the extravasation is detected during administration.

v. What is the organ target for cumulative dose toxicity for the particular drug?

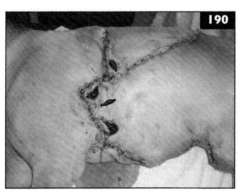

190 A large wound was closed using a single pedicle advancement flap and a photograph taken postoperatively (190).

i. What has been applied to the wound?

ii. Why has this procedure been performed?

iii. What are the benefits and potential complications?

189i. This dog has an approximately 2.3 cm full thickness skin wound and marked erythema surrounding the ulcer. The wound is on the mid antebrachium overlying the cephalic vein.
ii. This dog was diagnosed with osteosarcoma. The two most commonly used chemotherapeutics used to treat osteosarcoma are carboplatin/cisplatin and doxorubicin. Of these two drugs, doxorubicin is the more likely to have caused this wound because it is a powerful vesicant. Other chemotherapeutics that act as vesicants include vinca alkaloids. These drugs can cause extravasation-related phlebitis and associated tissue damage.
iii. This wound can be managed as an open wound. Debridement of necrotic tissue should be performed. Topical wound treatment and bandaging should be performed daily. An e-collar will be necessary to avoid further damage. Closure of the wound is contraindicated initially, because the necrosis could still be progressing, depending on the amount of doxorubicin that was extravasated.
iv. If the extravasation is detected, the placed IV catheter should be aspirated to remove as much of the drug as possible. Cold compresses can be applied topically. Dexrazoxane, an iron chelator, is recommended if extravasation has occurred. Treatment is recommended to occur as early as possible following extravasation (Venable, 2012). It can be administered both locally and systemically at 10 times the dose of doxorubicin.
v. Cumulative cardiac toxicity is expected after 180–240 mg/m^2.

190i. Medical leeches (*Hirudo medicinalis*) are applied to the wound.
ii. Venous congestion is a serious complication that can be associated with reconstructive surgery. Venous congestion occurs when venous outflow is decreased with respect to arterial inflow. Kinking of the relatively compliant veins or thrombus formation within the veins due to manipulation and movement of the skin can lead to venous congestion. Untreated venous congestion can lead to necrosis of the skin.
iii. Medical leeches are applied to the skin to remove excess venous blood until new microvasculature can form, preventing venous congestion. The saliva of leeches contains hiruden, a potent anticoagulant. The leeches drain blood directly by feeding and additionally, the location of the bite will continue to drain blood after the leech has detached. In small patients where loss of blood is a concern, a bandage can be placed following detachment of the leech. The leech is allowed to detach itself and is not forcefully detached from the tissue. Forceful detachment can lead to regurgitation of the normal flora of a leech's digestive tract. The leech contains *Aeromonas hydrophilia* within the digestive tract and regurgitation can lead to infection of the wound.

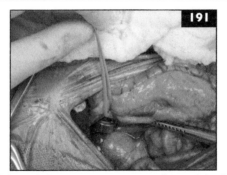

191 A 16-month-old Yorkshire Terrier presents for weight loss, polydipsia and polyuria, head pressing and abnormal behavior. Bloodwork shows low BUN, cholesterol, and albumin. Based on the signalment, clinical signs and bloodwork results you are suspicious of a portosystemic shunt.

i. What are the typical tests used for diagnosis?

ii. How is this process medically managed?

iii. Describe the surgical procedure pictured (**191**).

iv. After surgery, the patient develops seizures. How should this be managed?

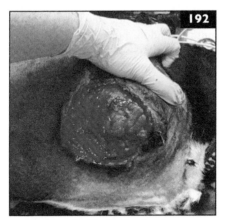

192 A 10-year-old neutered, male Pit Bull mix dog presented 3 days ago with a contaminated and necrotic wound, as a result of pressure necrosis following previous right mid-humeral amputation. The wound was dressed initially with honey. A healthy granulation bed is now present with a moderate to large amount of exudate (**192**). Calcium alginate is your dressing of choice.

i. What are the characteristics and properties of calcium alginate?

ii. What are the contraindications for its use? Why?

191i. Liver function tests, such as bile acids and resting ammonia levels, are useful as initial tests. In some cases, abdominal ultrasound can be used to identify the aberrant vessel. CT angiography and per-rectal or splenic scintigraphy using technetium are reliable ways of confirming the presence of the shunt.
ii. Medical management includes a low protein diet, oral lactulose to decrease the colonic absorption of ammonia and an oral antibiotic. Neomycin is a good choice because it is effective against the colonic bacteria without being systemically absorbed. In severe cases, lactulose/neomycin mixture may be administered as an enema.
iii. Ameroid constrictor application to a portocaval shunt.
iv. Postoperative seizures should be treated with the administration of a benzodiazepine, either diazepam or midazolam. If seizures recur, a constant rate infusion (CRI) of a benzodiazepine should be instituted. If the breakthrough seizures still occur, a propofol CRI should be instituted. Importantly, the patient should be started on a maintenance antiepileptic drug, preferably one that is not metabolized by the liver and is quick to reach steady state, such as levetiracetam.

192i. Calcium alginate is a non-occlusive, non-adhesive, hydrophilic, moisture retaining dressing derived from seaweed. Some of the properties include promotion of granulation tissue formation, epithelialization and hemostasis. Promotion of hemostasis is achieved due to the high calcium content of calcium alginate. Calcium alginate is indicated during transition from the inflammatory to repair phase of healing, especially when a large amount of exudate is present.
ii. This dressing should not be used in cases where little exudate is present, in addition to exposed muscle, tendon, bone or dry necrotic tissues. Usage in this situation causes adherence to underlying tissue and is contraindicated.

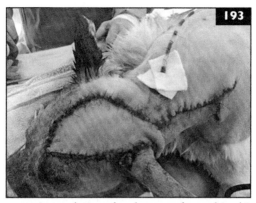

193 i. What reconstruction technique has been performed in this dog (193)?
ii. What are the anatomical landmarks for this technique?

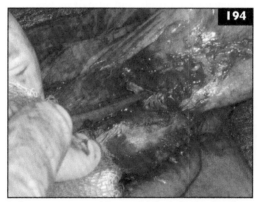

194 A photograph from a 1-year-old spayed female dog is shown (194). The dog had been spayed approximately 2 months previously. Approximately 1 month following the spay surgery, the dog had developed a wound with purulent drainage near the spay incision. The wound and drainage resolved with the administration of broad spectrum antibiotics. Approximately 1 month following the termination of antibiotic treatment, the wound returned.
i. What are the primary differential diagnoses for this draining wound?
ii. What diagnostic procedures would be performed?

193i. A caudal auricular axial pattern flap has been performed. This axial pattern flap is based on the sternocleidomastoid branches of the caudal auricular artery and vein.

ii. This axial pattern flap can be used to reconstruct the ear or dorsum of the head. The flap can extend rostrally to reconstruct defects overlying the orbit. The caudal auricular artery and vein are located in the palpable depression between the base of the auricular cartilage and the lateral aspect of the wing of the atlas. The skin flap base is centered over the lateral wing of the atlas. The dorsal and ventral landmarks extend as parallel lines in the central third of the cervical spine. The caudal margin of the flap is the level of the craniodorsal scapular spine.

194i. Differential diagnoses for a chronic draining tract include bacterial or fungal infection, foreign material, bony sequestra, neoplasia and osteomyelitis. Because of the history of a recent spay, a retained surgical sponge is considered likely. Drainage can also occur associated with non-absorbable sutures. Braided non-absorbable sutures have been reported to cause draining tracts in dogs. In this case, a surgical sponge was found and removed from the abdomen. Many adhesions were present and a thick fibrous capsule was found surrounding the surgical sponge.

ii. A CBC, serum biochemistry profile and urinalysis would be performed as a minimum database. The draining tract should be clipped and cleaned. A deep tissue culture and tissue biopsy should be obtained. Imaging of the abdomen should be performed. Some surgical sponges contain a radiopaque marker that is easily identified on radiographs and greatly aids in the diagnosis of retained sponge. In this case, a sponge containing a radiopaque marker was not used. If the radiopaque marker is not seen, a fistulogram or ultrasound examination could be considered. Fistulograms are reported to provide a definitive diagnosis of the cause of the draining tract in 58% of cases (Lamb, 1994). Surgical exploration of the abdomen can be recommended especially if the surgical report indicates that braided, non-absorbable suture was used in the spay or a retained surgical gauze is considered highly likely.

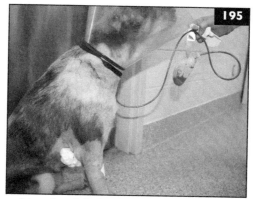

195 A wound created in a dog fight has been closed using delayed primary closure. Dead space was present when closure was accomplished. You decide to place a drain (**195**).
i. Define a closed, active drain.
ii. How will you decided when to remove this drain?
iii. List some potential reasons for drain failure.

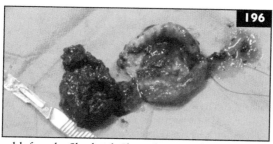

196 An 8-year-old female Shetland Sheepdog is admitted with signs of acute abdomen and icterus. On exploratory celiotomy a significantly distended, thickened gallbladder with black and green discoloration was found. A cholecystectomy is performed (**196**).
i. What is the diagnosis?
ii. What are the typical ultrasonographic findings of this disease?
iii. What are the treatment options?
iv. What is the prognosis following surgery and what factors are associated with a poor prognosis?

195i. A closed, active drain consists of tubing that is attached to a suction device. The suction will pull fluid through the fenestrations of the tube that are located within the lesion and from the tube into an external reservoir. The closed nature of the system will decrease infection risk and prevent damage to the skin due to draining fluid.

ii. Determination of the appropriate time for drain removal is dependent upon the quantity and nature of the fluid present, as well as the ongoing function of the drain. The longer a drain remains in place, the higher the risk of bacterial colonization. In healing tissue, the fluid within the drain should become increasingly serosanguineous and the amount of fluid produced should decrease until a plateau occurs. Frequent cytology can be performed to evaluate the presence of infection. Drain fluid production will rarely reach zero as the drain itself will induce a reaction by the body and the presence of active suction alters the balance of hydrostatic and oncotic pressures in the interstitial space.

iii. Drains may fail due to inappropriate tube diameter, improper positioning, the presence of tissue or blood clots within drain fenestrations, retrograde contamination or loss of suction.

196i. This dog has a biliary mucocele. While biliary mucocele can occur in any breed, Shetland Sheepdogs are over-represented.

ii. Ultrasonographic examination of the gallbladder usually reveals echogenic material within the gallbladder with a striated, stellate or mixed pattern known as 'kiwi fruit' pattern. Gallbladder rupture may also be visualized by the presence of lack of continuity of the gallbladder wall, pericholecystic hyperechoic fat and/or free abdominal fluid.

iii. Cholecystectomy is the surgical treatment of choice aiming at removing the source of excessive mucous production. In the presence of extrahepatic biliary obstruction, bile duct patency should be verified by catheterization and flushing.

iv. Some variability exists in the prognosis following surgery to treat biliary mucocele. In one study, the mortality rate associated with gallbladder mucocele was 32% if the gallbladder was not ruptured and 68% if the gallbladder was ruptured (Aguirre, 2007). The long-term prognosis for dogs with gallbladder mucocele is excellent if the patient survives for 2 weeks following surgery (Amsellem, 2006). Factors associated with a poor prognosis include elevated postoperative lactate concentrations and hypotension (Malek, 2013).

197 An intraoperative photograph is shown of a surgical procedure in progress (**197**). The surgeon is planning to use an axial pattern flap to close the defect.

i. The surgeon is planning an axial pattern flap based on what artery?

ii. Anatomically, where are the vessels supplying this flap located?

iii. What are two methods to allow the axial pattern flap to join the wound?

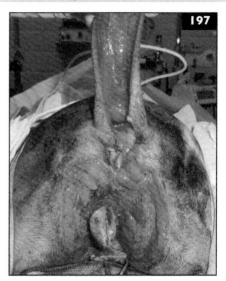

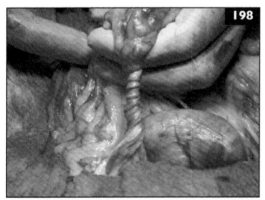

198 A 2-year-old male Collie with unilateral abdominal cryptorchidism is admitted with a history of abdominal pain associated with an abdominal mass. The dog underwent an exploratory celiotomy (**198**).

i. What is your diagnosis?

ii. What are the causes of this condition and how can a diagnosis be achieved?

iii. What is the treatment of this condition and what is the prognosis?

197i. The surgeon is planning a lateral caudal artery (tail) axial pattern flap. This flap requires an incision along either the dorsal or ventral aspect of the tail. The caudal vertebrae are dissected out while maintaining the blood supply to the skin. The tail is amputated at the base, leaving only skin. The skin can be used for wounds over the caudodorsal pelvis or perineum.

ii. The vessels supplying the skin of the tail are located on the lateral aspect of the tail. For the proximal portion of the tail, the arteries run along the ventral aspect of the transverse processes of the caudal vertebrae. In the distal tail, the vessels course dorsal to the transverse processes of the caudal vertebrae. The vessels are located in the subcutaneous tissue and dissection must be down to the deep tail fascia.

iii. Intact skin is present between this axial pattern flap and the wound. Two methods of joining the defect and the axial pattern flap are a bridging incision and tubing the flap. Tubing the flap consists of suturing the cut edges together in the area overlying intact skin. The bridging incision can be created by incising through the 'bridge' of skin located between the axial pattern flap and the defect.

198i. This dog has testicular torsion. More accurately, this condition can be referred to as torsion of the spermatic cord.

ii. Testicular torsion is more commonly seen in cryptorchid animals rather than these with scrotal testicles. An intra-abdominal testicle is more prone to torsion than an inguinal or scrotal testicle, possibly because of the greater intra-abdominal mobility of the testicle. The presence of testicular neoplasms associated with abdominally cryptorchid testicles may also predispose to testicular torsion. A tentative diagnosis of testicular torsion is based on history, clinical signs and diagnostic imaging findings. A palpable intra-abdominal mass in a cryptorchid dog, a decreased echogenicity of the testicle on ultrasound and an absent or decreased blood flow to and from the testicle on color Doppler all lead to a tentative diagnosis of testicular torsion. Definite diagnosis, however, is made with surgical abdominal exploration.

iii. Emergency surgical intervention is indicated to treat testicular torsion. Surgical excision of the affected testis should be performed and the prognosis is good. Concurrent surgical removal of a normal testis may be performed.

199 A lateral thoracic view of an angiogram (**199a**) is shown from a 6-month-old spayed, female Labrador Retriever with a grade V/VI left basilar continuous murmur. A lateral thoracic radiograph of the same dog is shown following treatment (**199b**).
i. What is your diagnosis?
ii. Correction of this defect can result in an acute decrease in the patient's heart rate. Explain.
iii. What congenital thoracic venous anomaly can interfere with surgical exposure when correcting this defect?
iv. What treatment was performed in this dog?

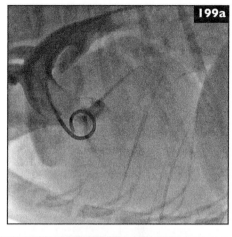

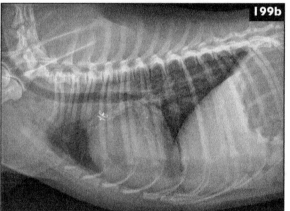

200 Hypoalbuminemia is often encountered in critically ill patients. During pre-operative bloodwork, a 25 kg mixed breed dog is noted to have an albumin of 1.0 g/dL.
i. For this patient, approximately what volume of plasma would be required to increase the albumin to 2.0 g/dL?
ii. Human albumin 25% can be utilized to increase albumin. What risks are associated with administration of this product?

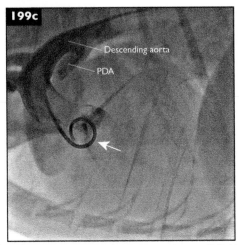

199i. A left to right shunting patent ductus arteriosus (PDA) is present. The catheter (arrow) in this image was inserted into the femoral artery and courses retrograde through the descending aorta and ascending aorta to the aortic root. The PDA is highlighted with contrast traveling from the descending aorta into the pulmonary artery (**199c**).

ii. An acute bradycardia can be associated with sudden occlusion of a PDA or arteriovenous fistula. This is commonly referred to as the 'Branham reflex'. It is thought to be related to vagal activation due to an increase in systemic blood pressure, which signals a reflex bradycardia via the high-pressure baroreceptors.

iii. Persistent left cranial vena cava. This is a normal vessel in the fetus that drains into the coronary sinus. In some animals it can persist but typically is of no clinical significance. Provided there is a normal right cranial vena cava, the persistent left cranial vena cava can be surgically ligated and divided. Alternatively, it can be isolated and gently retracted dorsally for visualization of the PDA.

iv. Transcatheter occlusion of the PDA has been performed with an Amplatz canine ductal occluder (ACDO) device.

200i. Approximately 30–45 mL/kg of plasma is required to increase albumin by 1.0 g/dL. This patient would require 750–1,125 mL of plasma to increase albumin to 2.0 g/dL.

ii. Anaphylactoid and type III (delayed) hypersensitivity reactions have been observed when human albumin has been administered to normal dogs, but adverse reactions in critically ill patients have been noted to be minimal. Hypertension has also been associated with albumin administration, so blood pressure should be monitored during the transfusion.

201 A 4-year-old castrated, male Labrador Retriever dog presents for a non-healing wound of several months duration. The owners originally noted the dog licking his paw excessively following a hunting trip. The dog will occasionally show signs of inter-mittent lameness on the affected limb; however, in general, normal activity is not affected. On physical examination there is soft tissue swelling, moderate-severe erythema and discomfort on palpation of the dorsal aspect of the left front paw. A draining tract on the surface is also apparent (201). Cytology of purulent–hemorrhagic exudate from the draining tract reveals numerous degenerate neutrophils and several macrophages. Organisms are not readily apparent.

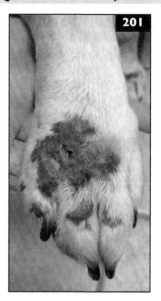

i. Based on the history and examination findings, what are your differential diagnoses for the lesion seen?
ii. What additional diagnostics are recommended for this patient?

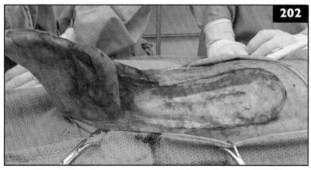

202 A reconstruction following mass removal is underway (202).
i. Name the reconstruction depicted.
ii. Name the artery and vein involved in this reconstruction method.
iii. Name four defect locations this method of reconstruction can be used to repair.

201i. Differentials include: infectious (bacterial; atypical bacteria including *Mycobacteria, Nocardia, Actinomyces* species; L-form infection; fungal – opportunistic, deep fungal mycoses including sporotrichosis, blastomycosis, coccidioidomycosis, histoplasmosis, cryptococcosis); inflammatory (foreign body reaction; sterile pyogranuloma/granuloma syndrome; trauma); neoplastic (mast cell tumor; cutaneous lymphoma; soft tissue sarcoma).

ii. Culture and susceptibility testing for bacterial (including atypical bacteria) and fungal organisms is warranted along with biopsy for histopathologic examination. Radiographs (or advanced imaging such as CT or MRI) would be helpful to determine whether underlying bony involvement is present or if there is the presence of foreign material. Contrast fistulogram may also be helpful for delineating the extent of the draining tract. If the lesion is due to a foreign body reaction (as was the case in the dog described – a lesion associated with migrating plant material), this may be beneficial for surgical planning and debridement of the wound.

202i. This is a caudal superficial epigastric axial pattern flap. This flap is raised from the caudal ventral abdomen including the caudal three or four mammary glands (dog) or second through fourth (cat). The medial border of this flap is the ventral midline of the animal. In male dogs, the base of the prepuce must be included in the flap in order to include the necessary vasculature. The distance between the ventral midline and the nipple is measured. This same distance is measured extending lateral to the nipple – identifying the lateral border. The flap is extended cranially between the first and second mammary glands, or shorter depending on need. Caudally, the flap remains intact to preserve its arterial supply and venous drainage. The mammary glands remain functional following relocation. Therefore, ovariohysterectomy may be recommended.

ii. This axial pattern flap is supplied by the caudal superficial epigastric artery and vein.

iii. This flap can be used to reconstruct skin defects located in the caudal abdomen, thigh, inguinal area, perineum, prepuce and rear limbs, as well as flank defects.

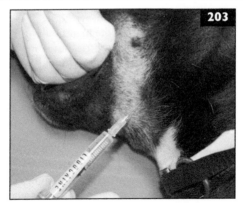

203 An 8-year-old intact Labrador Retriever mix presents for a partial right mandibulectomy to remove a squamous cell carcinoma localized cranial to the premolars. As part of the multimodal analgesia a local block (203) will be performed.
i. What is the name of the block?
ii. How is it performed?
iii. What area is desensitized?

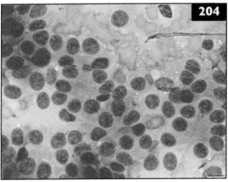

204 A fine-needle aspirate (FNA) of a mass associated with the anal sac of a dog is shown (204).
i. Given the cytologic appearance, what is your diagnosis?
ii. What is the most common site for this tumor to metastasize to?
iii. What is a possible related abnormality that can be seen on a chemistry panel?

Answers: 203, 204

203i. This block is a caudal inferior alveolar nerve block.

ii. This nerve is blocked at its entrance into the mandibular foramen using 0.2–0.5 ml/kg of local anesthetic. There are two approaches – intraoral and extraoral. The lingual surface of the mandible is palpated caudal and ventral to the last molar in an attempt to locate the mandibular foramen. Once the foramen has been identified, the intraoral technique involves passing a 25 mm, 25–27 gauge needle between the finger (guide) and the mandible in a ventrocaudal direction towards the angular process through the mucosa at the level of the last molar, until the foramen is reached where the local anesthetic is injected.

The extraoral technique entails localizing the mandibular foramen with a finger of the non-dominant hand. A needle is introduced through the skin at the level of the ventral notch of the mandible, cranial to the angular process and guided perpendicular to the ventral margin of the mandible toward the mandibular foramen between the mandible and the anesthetist's finger.

iii. This block provides analgesia for the buccal mucosa, mandibular teeth and lower lip. The mandibular branch (V3) of the central nerve V (trigeminal nerve) is blocked.

204i. Apocrine gland adenocarcinoma of the anal sac. The cytologic appearance of many bare nuclei in a 'sea' of cytoplasm with minimal anisokaryosis is typical of this tumor.

ii. Adenocarcinomas of the anal glands of the anal sac tend to metastasize (>50% of dogs present with metastases at the time of diagnosis [Hobson 2006]) to the medial iliac lymph nodes and can be diagnosed with FNA and cytologic examination.

iii. Approximately 25–90% (Hobson 2006) of dogs with adenocarcinoma of the anal glands of the anal sac will exhibit hypercalcemia, reflected by an elevated total calcium concentration. This paraneoplastic syndrome is usually mediated by production of parathyroid hormone-related peptide by neoplastic cells and is associated with a worse prognosis (Williams, 2003b).

205 An 11-year-old spayed, female Basset Hound presents for evaluation of sneezing with the recent development of epistaxis (unilateral, left sided). CBC, biochemistry and coagulation times are unremarkable. Blood pressure is 130 mmHg (systolic). A CT scan is performed under general anesthesia (**205**).

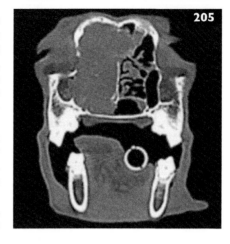

i. Based on the clinical description, what are the differential diagnoses? After reviewing the CT scan images, which differential diagnoses are considered to be most likely and why?

ii. When performing transnasal biopsies, which landmarks should be utilized to minimize potential complications?

iii. What are the current treatment recommendations for the most likely diagnoses in this case?

iv. During nasal biopsies, excessive hemorrhage occurs. Which techniques can be utilized to control bleeding?

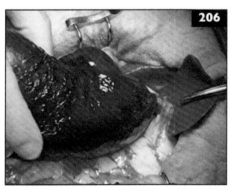

206 An intraoperative photograph is presented of the cranial abdomen at time of celiotomy in a 13-year- old castrated, male British Blue presenting for acute abdominal signs (**206**).

i. What is the diagnosis?

ii. What can be performed in the preoperative period to come to this diagnosis?

iii. What is the most common location for this condition in dogs?

Answers: 205, 206

205i. Neoplasia (adenocarcinoma is the most common nasal carcinoma in the dog), inflammatory rhinitis, infectious (fungal) rhinitis, foreign body and dental disease are appropriate initial differential diagnoses. Upon evaluation of CT images, due to the presence of bony destruction, neoplasia and infectious (fungal) rhinitis are considered to be more likely.

ii. Nasal biopsies can be collected using biopsy forceps, a plastic cannula/catheter or a bone curette. When utilizing the transnasal route, instruments should not be inserted past the level of the medial canthus of the eye, to avoid penetration of the cribriform plate.

iii. For most nasal tumors, fractionated radiation therapy is considered the treatment of choice. Surgical removal does not offer significant improvement in survival times when performed as the sole therapy, but may be useful in conjunction with radiation therapy. For nasal aspergillosis (fungal rhinitis), topical clotrimazole therapy is recommended if the cribriform plate is intact.

iv. If the animal has awakened from anesthesia, sedation should be administered. Nasal tamponade can be utilized for a short period of time. Application of cold pack can also be useful but is often not well tolerated in awake animals. Dilute epinephrine 1:100,000 can be applied topically using a cannula or packing soaked gauze into the nasal cavity. Rarely, hemorrhage cannot be controlled using these techniques, and ligation of the external carotid artery may be necessary.

206i. Liver lobe torsion.

ii. Color-flow Doppler ultrasonography can be helpful in detecting compromised blood flow to a specific liver lobe in cases suspected to have liver lobe torsion. However, ultrasound has poor sensitivity of detecting liver lobe margins when peritoneal fluid is not present. Contrast-enhanced CT can be helpful to provide a diagnosis of liver lobe torsion, as postcontrast images will show a lack of contrast within the torsed liver lobe.

iii. The left lateral liver lobe has been most commonly reported to undergo torsion in dogs. It has been suggested this is because of its large size and range of mobility and relative separation from other lobes. Liver masses have also been suggested to stretch ligamentous attachments to liver lobes allowing for increased mobility; however, this has not been substantiated in the veterinary literature.

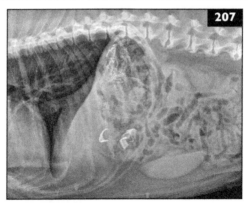

207 A 3-year-old Labrador Retriever is diagnosed with a gastric foreign body (**207**). The dog has a history of consuming a bandage 4 days prior. The dog has experienced severe vomiting for 1 day. A gastrotomy is planned.

i. What blood work abnormalities are expected?

ii. Describe the surgical procedure.

iii. What postoperative care should be provided?

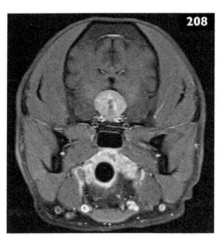

208 A 7-year-old Poodle is admitted for a chronic history of polyuria, polydipsia and polyphagia. Pyoderma is evident on physical exam, and endocrine testing is consistent with pituitary-dependent hyperadrenocorticism. A brain MRI is performed (**208**).

i. Name the surgical treatment for this disease process.

ii. What are the short-term risks and complications associated with this procedure?

iii. What are the long-term risks and complications?

207i. It is likely that this dog has dehydration, electrolyte abnormalities, and acid–base abnormalities due to severe vomiting for 1 day. Acute vomiting can lead to metabolic alkalosis because of a loss of gastric acid and chloride.

ii. A gastrotomy is performed through a standard ventral midline incision. The stomach is identified and isolated by placing stay sutures and by packing the stomach off from the other abdominal contents using laparotomy sponges. The gastrotomy incision is located in the center of the body between the branches of the gastric and gastroepiploic arteries. If the foreign body is fixed, the gastrotomy incision is located near the foreign object without damaging vital structures. Multiple stay sutures are placed around the proposed gastrotomy site. A stab incision is made with a scalpel blade and the incision is enlarged with scissors or a scalpel blade. Grasping or scooping instruments are used to locate and remove the foreign object. Prior to closing, the serosal surface is palpated to identify additional foreign material. The gastrotomy incision is closed in two layers: the first is a simple continuous pattern of 3-0 absorbable suture; the second is a continuous inverting pattern of 3-0 absorbable suture. The area is lavaged.

iii. Intraoperatively and following the gastrotomy procedure, the dog will need IV fluid administration. The IV fluid is selected based on electrolyte abnormalities and acid–base status. Water can be offered following surgery and food can be administered as small meals approximately 8–12 hours following surgery. Analgesics should be administered as needed.

208i. Trans-sphenoidal hypophysectomy.

ii. As with any surgery, there is the risk of hemorrhage. Due to the ventral approach and location of the arterial cerebral circle, accidental manipulation of the vasculature can lead to an arterial bleed. Keratoconjunctivitis sicca can be seen transiently after the procedure, but normal tear production should return within a few weeks.

iii. The most common long-term complication is diabetes insipidus. Since a complete hypophysectomy is performed, loss of circulating vasopressin is a result. Therefore, vasopressin may need to be supplemented in the form of desmopressin. Also, secondary hypothyroidism can be seen due to the pituitary gland's role in thyroid hormone regulation. Both of these complications may be permanent.

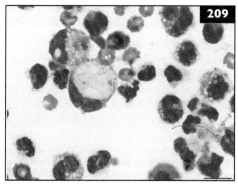

209 A direct smear prepared from peritoneal fluid aspirated from a 2-year-old spayed, female Dachshund is shown (**209**).
i. How would you classify the fluid?
ii. What are the most common causes of this type of abdominal effusion?
iii. How do you know that an enterocentesis was not performed?

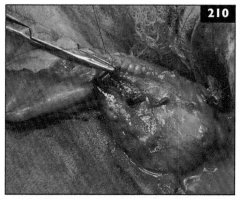

210 A 9-year-old male Poodle is diagnosed with extrahepatic biliary tract obstruction associated with chronic fibrosing pancreatitis.
i. Name the surgical procedure (**210**).
ii. What is the aim of surgery?
iii. What are the indications for performing this type of surgery?
iv. What are the complications?

209i. Septic suppurative exudate. Although a nucleated cell count is not given, knowing that this is a direct smear, the cell density is high and therefore the nucleated cell concentration of the fluid is increased. The sample is composed of a majority of moderately to markedly degenerate neutrophils, some of which contain a mixed population of phagocytozed bacteria.

ii. Septic suppurative exudates are most commonly due to penetration/rupture of a hollow viscus in the abdomen, although severe gastroenteritis, abscessation of the liver or prostate, chronic bile peritonitis and hematogenous spread of bacteria have also been reported.

iii. An enterocentesis would consist of a mixed population of bacteria without the presence of nucleated cells such as neutrophils, macrophages and mesothelial cells. In some instances, it can be difficult to determine whether the sample is the result of an acute rupture of intestines or an enterocentesis, although inflammation and translocation of bacteria leading to an exudate usually occur prior to tissue compromise severe enough to result in rupture of intestines.

210i. Pictured is a cholecystoduodenostomy underway.

ii. In the presence of extrahepatic biliary obstruction cholecystoenterostomy (cholecystoduodenostomy or cholecystojejunostomy) are used to establish bile duct patency by diverting bile from the gallbladder to the intestine. Either of these procedures allows bile to flow from the hepatic ducts into the gallbladder and then through a stoma created between the gallbladder and the duodenum/jejunum bypassing the common bile duct. The stoma between the two structures should be at least 4 cm in length. This wide opening allows any reflux moving from the small intestine into the gallbladder to be returned to the small intestine rather than becoming trapped in the biliary tract.

iii. Indications for performing cholecystoenterostomy include chronic fibrosing pancreatitis, neoplasia, trauma, cholelithiasis, abscessation and granuloma.

iv. Complications related to cholecystoenterostomy include stricture of the stoma, dehiscence of the anastomosis, cholangiohepatitis, hepatic abscess, acquired portosystemic shunts and pancreatitis (Papazoglou, 2008).

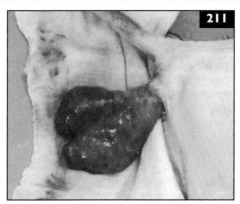

211 A 3-year-old female Persian cat presents after delivery of three kittens 2 hours previously. The perineal area is shown (**211**).
i. What is the diagnosis?
ii. Are there any predisposing factors?
iii. What are the treatment options and prognosis?

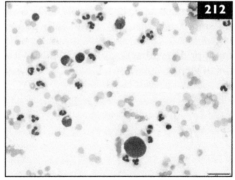

212 A direct smear prepared from peritoneal fluid obtained from a 6-year-old spayed, female Shetland Sheepdog is shown (**212**).
i. Is the cell count of the fluid elevated? What cells predominate?
ii. What two diagnostic tests should be performed on the fluid?
iii. What is the most common underlying disease or condition causing this effusion?

211i. The cat has a uterine prolapse. In this cat, both uterine horns and part of the uterine body have prolapsed.

ii. An open cervix is a prerequisite for the prolapse to take place; the condition is met during or after parturition. Most of the affected animals prolapse within 2 hours of delivery of their last kitten.

iii. Treatment may be surgical or medical and depends on the condition of the prolapsed uterus and the owner expectations associated with future reproduction of his cat. If the uterus is ulcerated and necrotic or the reduction of the prolapse is impossible, an amputation of the prolapsed uterus after ligation of the ovarian and uterine vessels is required. Manual reduction under general anesthesia or reduction and ovariohysterectomy through a midline celiotomy may be performed in a healthy uterus. Hemorrhage associated with rupture of the uterine or ovarian vessels should be managed with a blood transfusion and surgical reduction with ovariohysterectomy. Prognosis is usually good if treatment is provided promptly.

212i. Yes, the cell count of the fluid is elevated, and this is most likely an exudate. The light blue background indicates an elevated total protein concentration as well. The predominant cell is the mildly degenerate neutrophil; macrophages and reactive mesothelial cells are also present.

ii. Measurement of bilirubin concentration of the fluid and in the peripheral blood is recommended. If the bilirubin concentration of the fluid is greater than two times that of the blood, it is consistent with bile peritonitis. Bacterial culture and sensitivity are also recommended as approximately 50% of bile peritonitis cases are septic rather than sterile and this may result in a poorer prognosis for the patient (Mehler 2004).

iii. The most common primary diagnosis in patients with bile peritonitis is necrotizing cholecystitis (Mehler 2004).

References

Abelson AL, Armitage-Chan E, Lindsey JC, Wetmore LA. 2011. A comparison of epidural morphine with low dose bupivacaine versus epidural morphine alone on motor and respiratory function in dogs following splenectomy. *Veterinary Anaesthesia and Analgesia* **38**:213–223.

Aguirre AL, Center SA, Randolph JF, *et al.* 2007. Gallbladder disease in Shetland Sheepdogs: 38 cases (1995–2005). *Journal of the American Veterinary Medical Association* **231**:79–88.

Amsellem PM, Seim HB, MacPhail CM, *et al.* 2006. Long-term survival and risk factors associated with biliary surgery in dogs: 34 cases (1994–2004). *Journal of the American Veterinary Medical Association* **229**:1451–1457.

Anagnostou TL, Kazakos GM, Savvas I, Papazoglou LG, Rallis TS, Raptopoulos D. 2011. Remifentanil/isoflurane anesthesia in five dogs with liver disease undergoing liver biopsy. *Journal of the American Animal Hospital Association* **47**:103–109.

Anderson DM, Robinson RK, White RAS. 2000. Management of inflammatory polyps in 37 cats. *Veterinary Record* **147**:684–687.

Armbrust LJ, Biller DS, Bamford A, Chun R, Garrett LD, Sanderson MW. 2012. Comparison of three-view thoracic radiography and computed tomography for detection of pulmonary nodules in dogs with neoplasia. *Journal of the American Veterinary Medical Association* **240**:1088–1094.

Atkins C, Bonagura J, Ettinger S, *et al.* 2009. Guidelines for the diagnosis and treatment of canine chronic valvular heart disease. *Journal of Veterinary Internal Medicine* **23**:1142–1150.

Barrera JS, Bernard F, Ehrhart EJ, Withrow SJ, Monnet E. 2013. Evaluation of risk factors for outcome associated with adrenal gland tumors with or without invasion of the caudal vena cava and treated via adrenalectomy in dogs: 86 cases (1993–2009). *Journal of the American Veterinary Medical Association* **242**:1715–1721.

Beck AL, Grierson JM, Ogden DM, Hamilton MH, Lipscomb VJ. 2007. Outcome of and complications associated with tube cystostomy in dogs and cats: 76 cases (1995–2006). *Journal of the American Veterinary Medical Association* **230**:1184–1189.

Becker WM, Beal M, Stanley BJ, Hauptman JG. 2012. Survival after surgery for tracheal collapse and the effect of intrathoracic collapse on survival. *Veterinary Surgery* **41**(4):501–506.

Berent AC, Weisse C, Beal MW, Brown DC, Todd K, Bagley D. 2011. Use of indwelling, double-pigtail stents for treatment of malignant ureteral obstruction in dogs: 12 cases (2006–2009). *Journal of the American Veterinary Medical Association* **238**:1017–1025.

Berent AC, Weisse C, Mayhew PD, Todd K, Wright M, Bagley D. 2012. Evaluation of cystoscopic-guided laser ablation of intramural ectopic ureters in female dogs. *Journal of the American Veterinary Medical Association* **240**:716–725.

References

Bhandal J, Kuzma A. 2008. Tracheal rupture in a cat: Diagnosis by computed tomography. *Canadian Veterinary Journal* **49**:595–597.

Bonfanti U, Bertazzolo W, Bottero E, *et al.* 2006. Diagnostic value of cytologic examination of gastrointestinal tract tumors in dogs and cats: 83 cases (2001–2004). *Journal of the American Veterinary Medical Association* **229**:1130–1133.

Boothe HW, Howe LM, Boothe DM, Reynolds LA, Carpenter M. 2010. Evaluation of outcomes in dogs treated for pyothorax: 46 cases (1983–2001). *Journal of the American Veterinary Medical Association* **236**:657–663.

Boston SE, Higginson G, Monteith G. 2011. Concurrent splenic and right atrial mass at presentation in dogs with HAS: a retrospective study. *Journal of the American Animal Hospital Association* **47**:336–341.

Burns CG, Bergh MS, McLaughlin MA. 2013. Surgical and nonsurgical treatment of peritoneopericardial diaphragmatic hernia in dogs and cats: 58 cases (1999–2008). *Journal of the American Veterinary Medical Association* **242**:643–650.

Cannizzo KL, McLoughlin MA, Mattoon JS, Samii VF, Chew DJ, DiBartola SP. 2003. Evaluation of transurethral cystoscopy and excretory urography for diagnosis of ectopic ureters in female dogs: 25 cases (1992–2000). *Journal of the American Veterinary Medical Association* **223**:475–481.

Culp WTN, Ehrhart N, Withrow SJ, *et al.* 2013. Results of surgical excision and evaluation of factors associated with survival time in dogs with lingual neoplasia: 97 cases (1995–2008). *Journal of the American Veterinary Medical Association* **242**:1392–1397.

Dvorak LD, Beaver DP, Ellison GW, Bellah JR, Mann FA, Henry CJ. 2004. Major glossectomy in dogs: a case series and proposed classification system. *Journal of the American Animal Hospital Association* **40**:331–337.

Ellison GW. 2004. Alapexy: an alternative technique for repair of stenotic nares in dogs. *Journal of the American Animal Hospital Association* **40**:484–489.

Gaastra W, Lipman LJA, De Cock AWAM, *et al.* 2010. *Pythium insidiosum*: an overview. *Veterinary Microbiology* **146**:1–16.

Gagnon D, Brisson B. 2013. Predisposing factors for colonic torsion/volvulus in dogs: a retrospective study of six cases (1992–2010). *Journal of the American Animal Hospital Association* **49**:169–174.

Gines JA, Friend EJ, Vives MA, Browne WJ, Tarlton JF, Chanoit G. 2011.Mechanical comparison of median sternotomy closure in dogs using polydioxanone and wire sutures. *Journal of Small Animal Practice* **52**:582–586.

Goldfinch N, Argyle D. 2012. Feline lung-digit syndrome: unusual metastatic patterns of primary lung tumours in cats. *Journal of Feline Medicine and Surgery* **14**:202–208.

Grimes JA, Schmiedt CW, Cornell KK, Radlinsk MG. 2011. Identification of risk factors for septic peritonitis and failure to survive following gastrointestinal surgery in dogs. *Journal of the American Veterinary Medical Association* 238:486–494.

Hammel SP, Bjorling DE. 2002. Results of vulvoplasty for treatment of recessed vulva in dogs. *Journal of the American Animal Hospital Association* 38:79–83.

Hardie EM, Spodnick GJ, Gilson SD, Benson JA, Hawkins EC. 1999. Tracheal rupture in cats: 16 cases (1983–1998). *Journal of the American Veterinary Medical Association* 214:508–512.

Hardie EM, Linder KE, Pease AP. 2008. Aural cholesteatoma in twenty dogs. *Veterinary Surgery* 37:763–770.

Harran NX, Bradley KJ, Hetzel N, Bowlt KL, Day MJ, Barr F. 2012. MRI findings of a middle ear cholesteatoma in a dog. *Journal of the American Animal Hospital Association* 48:339–343.

Herrera MA, Mehl ML, Kass PH, Pascoe PJ, Feldman EC, Nelson RW. 2008. Predictive factors and the effect of phenoxybenzamine on outcome in dogs undergoing adrenalectomy for pheochromocytoma. *Journal of Veterinary Internal Medicine* 22:1333–1339.

Hobson HP, Brown MR, Rogers KS. 2006. Surgery of metastatic anal sac adenocarcinoma in five dogs. *Veterinary Surgery* 35:267–270.

Huck JL, Stanley BJ, Hauptman JG. 2008. Technique and outcome of nares amputation (Trader's technique) in immature shih tzus. *Journal of the American Animal Hospital Association* 44: 82–85.

Kaufman KL, Mann FA. 2013. Short-and long-term outcomes after digit amputation in dogs: 33 cases (1999–2011). *Journal of the American Veterinary Medical Association* 242:1249–1254.

Keir I, Woolford L, Hirst C, Adamantos S. 2010. Fatal aortic oesophageal fistula following oesophageal foreign body removal in a dog. *Journal of Small Animal Practice* 51:657–660.

Kelly SE, Clark WT. 1995. Surgical repair of fracture of the os penis in a dog. *Journal of Small Animal Practice* 36:507–509.

Kirsch JA, Hauptman JG, Walshaw R. 2002. A Urethropexy technique for surgical treatment of urethral prolapse in the male dog. *Journal of the American Animal Hospital Association* 38: 381–384.

Kyles AE, Hardie EM, Wooden BG, *et al.* 2005. Management and outcome of cats with ureteral calculi: 153 cases (1984–2002). *Journal of the American Veterinary Medical Association* 226:937–944.

Lamb CR, White RN, McEvoy FJ. 1994. Sinography in the investigation of draining tracts in small animals: retrospective review of 25 cases. *Veterinary Surgery* 23:129–134.

References

Lanz O, Ellison GW, Bellah JR. 2001. Surgical treatment of septic peritonitis without abdominal drainage in 28 dogs. *Journal of the American Animal Hospital Association* 37:87–92.

Lascelles BD, Henderson RA, Seguin B, Liptak JM, Withrow SJ. 2004. Bilateral rostral maxillectomy and nasal planectomy for large rostral maxillofacial neoplasms in six dogs and one cat. *Journal of the American Animal Hospital Association* 40:137–146.

Lipscomb VJ, Hardie RJ, Dubielzig RR. 2003. Spontaneous pneumothorax caused by pulmonary blebs and bullae in 12 dogs. *Journal of the American Animal Hospital Association* 39:435–445.

Liptak JM, Dernell WS, Monnet E, *et al.* 2004. Massive hepatocellular carcinoma in dogs: 48 cases (1992–2002). *Journal of the American Veterinary Medical Association* 225:1225–1230.

Liptak JM, Kamstock DA, Dernell WS, Monteith GJ, Rizzo SA, Withrow SJ. 2008. Oncologic outcome after curative-intent treatment in 39 dogs with primary chest wall tumors (1992–2005). *Veterinary Surgery* 37:488–496.

Low WW, Uhl JM, Kass PH, Ruby AL, Westropp JL. 2010. Evaluation of trends in urolith composition and characteristics of dogs with urolithiasis: 25,499 cases (1985–2006). *Journal of the American Veterinary Medical Association* 236:193–200.

Mai W. 2006. The hilar perivenous hyperechoic triangle as a sign of acute splenic torsion in dogs. *Veterinary Radiology and Ultrasound* 47:487–491.

Malek S, Sinclair E, Hosgood G, Moens NMM, Baily T, Boston SE. 2013. Clinical findings and prognostic factors for dogs undergoing cholecystectomy for gall bladder mucocele. *Veterinary Surgery* 42:418–426.

Medl N, Guerrero TG, Holzele L, Hassig M, Lochbrunner S, Montavon PM. 2012. Intraoperative contamination of the suction tip in clean orthopedic surgeries in dogs and cats. *Veterinary Surgery* 41:254–260.

Mehler SJ, Mayhew PD, Drobatz KJ, Hold DE. 2004. Variables associated with outcome in dogs undergoing extrahepatic biliary surgery: 60 cases (1988–2002). *Veterinary Surgery* 33:644–649.

Millis DK, Nemzek J, Riggs C, Walshaw R. 1995. Gastric dilatation-volvulus after splenic torsion in two dogs. *Journal of the American Veterinary Medical Association* 207:314.

Mitchell SL, McCarthy R, Rudloff E, Pernell RT. 2000. Tracheal rupture associated with intubation in cats: 20 cases (1996–1998). *Journal of the American Veterinary Medical Association* 216:1592–1595.

Mittleman E, Weisse C, Mehler SJ, Lee JA. 2004. Fracture of an endoluminal nitinol stent used in the treatment of tracheal collapse in a dog. *Journal of the American Veterinary Medical Association* 225:1217–1221.

Murphy KA, Brisson BA. 2006. Evaluation of lung lobe torsion in pugs: 7 cases (1991–2004). *Journal of the American Veterinary Medical Association* **228**:86–90.

Neath PJ, Brockman DJ, King LG. 2000. Lung lobe torsion in dogs: 22 cases (1981–1999). *Journal of the American Veterinary Medical Association* **217**:1041–1044.

Neihaus SA, Hathcock TL, Boothe DM, Goring RL. 2011. Presurgical antiseptic efficacy of chlorhexidine diacetate and povidone-iodine in the canine prepucial cavity. *Journal of the American Animal Hospital Association* **47**:406–412.

Nelson DA, Miller MW, Gordon SG, Saunders A, Fossum TW. 2012. Minimally invasive transxiphoid approach to the cardiac apex and caudoventral intrathoracic space. *Veterinary Surgery* **41**:915–917.

Ouellet M, Dunn ME, Lussier B, Chailleux N, Helie P. 2006. Noninvasive correction of a fractured endoluminal nitinol tracheal stent in a dog. *Journal of the American Animal Hospital Association* **42**:467–471.

Papazoglou LG, Mann FA, Wagner-Mann C, Song KJE. 2008. Long-term survival of dogs after cholecystoenterostomy: a retrospective study of 15 cases (1981–2005). *Journal of the American Animal Hospital Association* **44**:67–74.

Patsikas MN, Rallis T, Kladakis SE, Dessiris AK. 2001. Computed tomography diagnosis of isolated splenic torsion in a dog. *Veterinary Radiology and Ultrasound* **42**:235–237.

Peterson ME. 2006. Snake bite: pit vipers. *Clinical Techniques in Small Animal Practice* **21**:174–182.

Rallis TS, Papazoglou LG, Adamama-Moraitou KK, Prassinos NN. 2000. Acute enteritis or gastroenteritis in young dogs as a predisposing factor for intestinal intussusception: a retrospective study. *Journal of Veterinary Medicine* **47**:507–511.

Rawlings CA, Bjorling DE, Christie BA. 2003. Kidneys. In: Slatter D (ed). *Textbook of Small Animal Surgery*, 3rd edn. Saunders, Philadelphia, pp. 1608–1609.

Risselada M, deRooster H, Liuti T, Polis I, van Bree H. 2006. Use of internal splinting to realign a noncompliant sternum in a cat with pectus excavatum. *Journal of the American Veterinary Medical Association* **228**:1047–1052.

Risselada M, Ellison GW, Bacon NJ, *et al.* 2010. Comparison of 5 surgical techniques for partial liver lobectomy in the dog for intraoperative blood loss and surgical time. *Veterinary Surgery* **39**:856–862.

Robbins MA, Mullen HS. 1994. En bloc ovariohysterectomy as a treatment for dystocia in dogs and cats. *Veterinary Surgery* **23**:48–52.

Schmide K, Bertani C, Martano M, Morello E, Buracco P. 2005. Reconstruction of the lower eyelid by third eyelid lateral advancement and local transposition cutaneous flap after 'en bloc' resection of squamous cell carcinoma in 5 cats. *Veterinary Surgery* **34**:78–82.

References

Schultz RM, Johnson EG, Wisner ER, Brown NA, Byrne BA, Sykes JE. 2008. Clinicopathologic and diagnostic imaging characteristics of systemic aspergillosis in 30 dogs. *Journal of Veterinary Internal Medicine* **22**:851–859.

Spivack RE, Elkins AD, Moore GE, Lantz GC. 2013. Postoperative complications following TECA-LBO in the dog and cat. *Journal of the American Animal Hospital Association* **49**:160–168.

Staatz AJ, Monnet E, Seim HB. 2002. Open peritoneal drainage versus primary closure for the treatment of septic peritonitis in dogs and cats: 42 cases (1993–1999). *Veterinary Surgery* **31**:174–180.

Stanley BJ, Hauptman JG, Fritz MC, Rosenstein DS, Kinns J. 2010. Esophageal dysfunction in dogs with idiopathic laryngeal paralysis: a controlled cohort study. *Veterinary Surgery* **39**:139–149.

Steckel RR. 2011. Use of an inguinal approach adapted from equine surgery for cryptorchidectomy in dogs and cats: 26 cases (1999–2010). *Journal of the American Veterinary Medical Association* **239**:1098–1103.

Stefanello D, Avallone G, Ferrari R, Roccabianca P, Boracchi, P. 2011. Canine cutaneous perivascular wall tumors at first presentation: clinical behavior and prognostic factors in 55 cases. *Journal of Veterinary Internal Medicine* **25**:1398–1405.

Stepnik MW, Mehl ML, Hardie EM, et al. 2009. Outcome of permanent tracheostomy for treatment of upper airway obstruction in cats: 21 cases (1990–2007). *Journal of the American Veterinary Medical Association* **234**:638–643.

Stone EA, Robertson JL, Metcalf MR. 2002. The effect of nephrotomy on renal function and morphology in dogs. *Veterinary Surgery* **31**:391–397.

Sturgeon C, Lamport AI, Lloyd DH, Muri P. 2000. Bacterial contamination of suction tips used during surgical procedures performed on dogs and cats. *American Journal of Veterinary Research* **61**:779–783.

Sura PA, Krahwinkel DJ. 2008. Self-expanding nitinol stents for the treatment of tracheal collapse in dogs: 12 cases (2001–2004). *Journal of the American Veterinary Medical Association* **232**:228–236.

Thieman KM, Krahwinkel DJ. 2010. Histopathological confirmation of polyneuropathy in 11 dogs with laryngeal paralysis. *Journal of the American Animal Hospital Association* **46**:161–167.

Thieman KM, Kirkby KA, Flynn-Lurie A, Grooters AM, Bacon NJ. 2011. Diagnosis and treatment of truncal cutaneous pythiosis in a dog. *Journal of the American Veterinary Medical Association* **239**:1232–1235.

Thompson HC, Cortes Y, Gannon K, Bailey D, Freer S. 2012. Esophageal foreign bodies in dogs: 34 cases (2004–2009). *Journal of Veterinary Emergency and Critical Care* **22**:253–261.

Tobias KM. 2007. Surgical stapling devices in veterinary medicine: a review. *Veterinary Surgery* **36**:341–349.

Trostel CT, Frankel DJ. 2010. Punch resection alaplasty technique in dogs and cats with stenotic nares: 14 cases. *Journal of the American Animal Hospital Association* **46**:5–11.

Venable RO, Saba CF, Endicott MM, Northrup NC. 2012. Dexrazoxane treatment of doxorubicin extravasation injury in four dogs. *Journal of the American Veterinary Medical Association* **240**:304–307.

Weisse CW, Berent AC, Todd KL, Solomon JA. 2008. Potential applications of interventional radiology in veterinary medicine. *Journal of the American Veterinary Medical Association* **233**:1564–1574.

Westropp JL, Ruby AL, Campbell SJ, Ling GV. 2010. Canine and feline urolithiasis: pathophysiology, epidemiology and management. In: Bojrab MJ, Monnet E (eds). *Mechanisms of Disease in Small Animal Surgery*, 3rd edn. Teton NewMedia, Jackson, WY pp. 388–389.

White RN. 2012. Surgical management of laryngeal collapse associated with brachycephalic airway obstruction syndrome in dogs. *Journal of Small Animal Practice* **53**:44–50.

Williams LE, Packer RA. 2003a. Association between lymph node size and metastasis in dogs with oral malignant melanoma: 100 cases (1987–2001). *Journal of the American Veterinary Medical Association* **222**:1234–1236.

Williams LE, Gliatto JM, Dodge RK, *et al.* 2003b. Carcinoma of the apocrine glands of the anal sac in dogs: 113 cases (1985–1995). *Journal of the American Veterinary Medical Association* **223**:825–831.

Williams JM, Sale CSH. 2006. Results of transthoracic esophagotomy retrieval of esophageal foreign body obstruction in dogs: 14 cases (2000–2004). *Journal of the American Animal Hospital Association* **42**:450–456.

Yates D, Hayes G, Heffernan M, Beynon R. 2003. Incidence of cryptorchidism in dogs and cats. *Veterinary Record* **152**:502–504.

Zikes C, McCarthy T. 2012. Bilateral ventriculocordectomy via ventral laryngotomy for idiopathic laryngeal paralysis in 88 dogs. *Journal of the American Animal Hospital Association* **48**:234–244.

Index

Note: references are to case numbers

218

Index

Index

Index

Index

Printed and bound by CPI Group (UK) Ltd, Croydon, CR0 4YY

23/10/2024

01777696-0001